# Radiofrequency Ablation for Small Hepatocellular Carcinoma

AF147621

Minshan Chen   •   Yaojun Zhang
Wan Y. Lau

**Editors**

# Radiofrequency Ablation for Small Hepatocellular Carcinoma

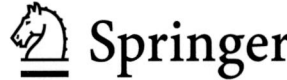 Springer

*Editors*
Minshan Chen
Department of Hepatobiliary Surgery
Sun Yat-sen University Cancer Center
Guangzhou
China

Yaojun Zhang
Department of Hepatobiliary Surgery
Sun Yat-sen University Cancer Center
Guangzhou
China

Wan Y. Lau
Academician of the
Chinese Academy of Sciences
Faculty of Medicine
The Chinese University of Hong Kong
Hong Kong SAR
China

ISBN 978-94-024-1323-6      ISBN 978-94-017-7258-7   (eBook)
DOI 10.1007/978-94-017-7258-7

Springer Dordrecht Heidelberg New York London

© Springer Science+Business Media Dordrecht 2016
Softcover re-print of the Hardcover 1st edition 2016
This work is subject to copyright. All rights are reserved by the Publisher, whether the whole or part of the material is concerned, specifically the rights of translation, reprinting, reuse of illustrations, recitation, broadcasting, reproduction on microfilms or in any other physical way, and transmission or information storage and retrieval, electronic adaptation, computer software, or by similar or dissimilar methodology now known or hereafter developed.
The use of general descriptive names, registered names, trademarks, service marks, etc. in this publication does not imply, even in the absence of a specific statement, that such names are exempt from the relevant protective laws and regulations and therefore free for general use.
The publisher, the authors and the editors are safe to assume that the advice and information in this book are believed to be true and accurate at the date of publication. Neither the publisher nor the authors or the editors give a warranty, express or implied, with respect to the material contained herein or for any errors or omissions that may have been made.

Printed on acid-free paper

Springer Science+Business Media B.V. Dordrecht is part of Springer Science+Business Media (www.springer.com)

# Preface

Hepatocellular carcinoma (HCC) is the fifth most common cancer in the world and the third most common cause of cancer-related deaths with about 600,000 patients dying from the disease annually. The incidence of HCC has been on the rise and is associated with an increase in hepatitis B- or C-associated cirrhosis.

Radiofrequency ablation (RFA) was introduced as a new treatment modality for HCC in the early 1990s. After several decades' development, RFA has been regarded as a representative modality of locoregional therapy because of its effectiveness and safety for small HCC (sHCC). Extensive studies have indicated that RFA has an outcome equal to that of surgical resection for sHCC, but has the advantage in being less invasive over surgical resection. However, the outcomes after RFA are largely dependent on the experience of operators, which is called "learning curve." On the other hand, operators from different departments (e.g., the departments of surgery, radiology, gastroenterology, oncology, and so on) usually have different opinions and experiences. It is important to standardize and generalize the procedures of RFA.

This will be the first book that focuses on RFA for sHCC. In this book, we firstly present the characteristics of sHCC and discuss why sHCC is the best candidate for RFA. Then we demonstrate all types of RFA systems which are commercially available, and their working principles, advantages, disadvantages, and so on. Following that, we show how to do RFA under the guidance of ultrasound, CT, laparoscopy, or during open operation. Finally, we discuss the radiologic assessment and follow up after RFA, as well as adjuvant therapies and clinical trials about RFA. It provides the most updated knowledge in the rapidly advancing field of RFA. Controversial areas are discussed by highly regarded authorities who look at the problem from different perspectives. And there is an extensive use of diagrams, figures, and tables to make the text easy to read.

The authors are from different departments, including the departments of pathology, radiology, surgery, and gastroenterology, as well as manufacturers. With this book, readers would have a clear idea on who, when, and how to do RFA. We aim to standardize and generalize the procedure of RFA, which will help to improve the outcomes of RFA for sHCC.

The intended readers of this book are clinicians who are interested in HCC or RFA, including liver surgeons, interventional and diagnostic radiologists, gastroenterologists, oncologists, and hepatologists. General physicians, general surgeons, trainees, hospital administrators, and instrument manufacturers will also find this book useful as a reference.

Guangzhou, China                                                         Minshan Chen

# Acknowledgements

I am deeply indebted to the contributions of the authors who have helped to bring together this volume of information on this important subject. I would like to acknowledge the indebtedness in particular to WanYee Lau, without whose unflagging help, encouragement, and personal efforts, the publication of this book would not have been possible.

I am grateful to Mr. James Hu from Springer Beijing who believed that a comprehensive book that focuses on radiofrequency ablation for small hepatocellular carcinoma was needed, and thank him for his great help with dedication and professionalism to this project.

Minshan Chen

# Contents

# Contributors

**Ashwin Kumar Bholee, MBBS** Department of Hepatobiliary Surgery, Sun Yat-sen University Cancer Center, Guangzhou, China

**Minshan Chen, MD, PhD** Department of Hepatobiliary Surgery, Sun Yat-sen University Cancer Center, Guangzhou, China

**Wenming Cong, MD, PhD** Department of Pathology, Eastern Hepatobiliary Surgery Hospital, Second Military Medical University, Shanghai, China

**Tamara Gall, MD, FRCS** Department of Surgery and Cancer, Hammersmith Campus, Imperial College London, London, UK

**Hengjun Gao, MD, PhD** Department of Hepatobiliary Surgery, Sun Yat-sen University Cancer Center, Guangzhou, China

**Long R. Jiao, MD, FRCS** Department of Surgery and Cancer, Hammersmith Campus, Imperial College London, London, UK

**Ming Kuang, MD, PhD** Department of Hepatobiliary Surgery, The First Affiliated Hospital of Sun Yat-sen University, Guangzhou, China

**Eric C.H. Lai, MBChB(CUHK), MRCS(Ed), FRACS** Department of Surgery, Pamela Youde Nethersole Eastern Hospital, Hong Kong SAR, China

**Stephanie H.Y. Lau, MBChB(CUHK), MRCS(Ed), FRCS(Ed)** Department of Surgery, Queen Elizabeth Hospital, Hong Kong SAR, China

**Wan Yee Lau, MD, DSc, FACS, FRCS, FRACS(Hon)** Academician of the Chinese Academy of Sciences, Faculty of Medicine, The Chinese University of Hong Kong, Shatin, New Territories, Hong Kong SAR, China

**Xinyuan Lu, MD** Department of Pathology, Eastern Hepatobiliary Surgery Hospital, Second Military Medical University, Shanghai, China

**Zhenwei Peng, MD, PhD** Department of Oncology, The First Affiliated Hospital of Sun Yat-sen University, Guangzhou, China

**Zoe Thompson, MD, FRCS** Department of Surgery and Cancer, Hammersmith Campus, Imperial College London, London, UK

**Yaojun Zhang, MD, PhD** Department of Hepatobiliary Surgery,
Sun Yat-sen University Cancer Center, Guangzhou, China

**Zhongguo Zhou, MD, PhD** Department of Hepatobiliary Surgery,
Sun Yat-sen University Cancer Center, Guangzhou, China

# Diagnosis of Small Hepatocellular Carcinoma

**1**

Ashwin Kumar Bholee and Minshan Chen

## 1.1 Introduction

Hepatocellular carcinoma (HCC) is the third most common malignancy worldwide and the second leading cause of cancer-related deaths [1]. Globally, there are approximately 750,000 new cases of liver cancer reported each year. Consensus guidelines have been published by different organizations, including the American Association for the Study of Liver Disease (AASLD), National Comprehensive Cancer Network (NCCN), and European Association for the Study of the Liver (EASL) to standardize the approach for diagnosis and treatment [2–4]. HCC is more effectively treated when it is diagnosed at an early stage, and the best chance for early diagnosis comes from surveillance of patients known to be at high risk. This includes patients with cirrhosis from any cause and carriers of hepatitis B or C [3]. The 2012 NCCN guidelines recommend screening high-risk patients with serum *a-fetoprotein* (AFP) and liver ultrasound (US) every 6 months to 12 months. A rising AFP associated with a liver nodule measuring larger than 1 cm raises suspicion for HCC and warrants evaluation with cross-sectional imaging [3]. The tests used to diagnose HCC include radiology, biopsy, and AFP serology. The diagnosis of HCC based on imaging can be challenging because of the imaging characteristics of a background of liver cirrhosis. A CT or MRI scan should be performed in cirrhotic patients with an ultrasound showing a lesion of > 1 cm, an elevated or rising AFP in the absence of a liver lesion on US, or when there is a clinical suspicion for the presence of HCC.

## 1.2 Role of AFP in Diagnosis

Alpha-fetoprotein has long been used for the diagnosis of HCC. It has also been part of surveillance algorithms. However, the AFP is insufficiently sensitive or specific for use as a surveillance assay. Recent data also suggest that its use as a diagnostic test is less specific than was once thought. AFP can be elevated in intrahepatic cholangiocarcinoma (ICC) and in some metastases from colorectal cancer [5, 6]. Therefore, the finding of a mass in the liver with an elevated AFP does not automatically indicate HCC. Since AFP can be elevated in either condition, the diagnosis of HCC must rest on radiological appearances and/or on histology.

## 1.3 Radiological Diagnosis of HCC

HCC can be diagnosed radiologically, without biopsy if the typical imaging features are present [7–14]. A contrast-enhanced cross-sectional scan

A.K. Bholee, MBBS • M. Chen (✉)
Department of Hepatobiliary Surgery, Sun Yat-sen University Cancer Center, Guangzhou, China
e-mail: chminsh@mail.sysu.edu.cn

© Springer Science+Business Media Dordrecht 2016
M. Chen et al. (eds.), *Radiofrequency Ablation for Small Hepatocellular Carcinoma*,
DOI 10.1007/978-94-017-7258-7_1

is required (dynamic CT scan or MR). HCC enhances more intensely in arterial phase. The blood supply of HCC mainly comes from the artery, whereas the arterial blood in the liver is diluted by venous blood that does not contain contrast. In the venous phase, HCC enhances less than the surrounding liver, as HCC does not have a portal blood supply and the arterial blood flowing through the lesion no longer contains contrast, whereas the portal blood in the liver contains contrast now. This is the so-called washout. In some cases, the presence of "washout" persists; however, sometimes, "washout" is only present in the delayed phase. This radiologic feature, arterial enhancement followed by portal washout, is highly specific for HCC [12, 13, 15]. Thus, a four-phase study is necessary to properly document the existence of HCC: unenhanced, arterial, venous, and delayed phases.

Forner et al. [15] used contrast ultrasound and MRI to evaluate lesions smaller than 2 cm found on surveillance. The positive predictive value of performing these two tests was 100 %, although the negative predictive value was about 42 %. It means that if both tests were positive, the lesion was always HCC. However, if one or both tests were not conclusive, then the false-negative detection rate of HCC was higher than 50 %. Under these circumstances, a biopsy may be performed. In this study, up to three biopsies were performed in an attempt to get the correct diagnosis. Another study came to similar conclusions [16] providing external validation of the algorithm. A third study [17], presented so far only as abstract, used CT scanning as well as contrast ultrasound and MRI also validated the algorithm. Using a single contrast-enhanced modality could have a lower positive predictive value than using two studies, although the positive predictive value was still better than 90 %. Although other studies have provided external validation of these algorithms, they have also shown that typical appearances of arterial enhance and venous washout are so highly specific that only a single study is necessary when these appearances are present [17, 18]. The sensitivity of using dual imaging was between 21 % and 37 %, and specificity was 100 % for diagnosis. In addition, two

studies now have shown that sequential imaging can be used to decrease the biopsy [17, 18]. Using sequential studies rather than requiring two studies to be typical improved the sensitivity to about 74–80 %, while the specificity fell to 89–97 %. A recent study has also shown that intrahepatic cholangiocarcinoma (ICC) does not show washout in the venous delayed phases at MRI, further stressing the specificity of this profile at early stages [19]. Additionally, false positives for HCC have been described for contrast-enhanced ultrasound in patients with biopsy proven ICC [20]. If there is any discrepancy between imaging techniques, a biopsy should be performed if treatment is to be considered.

Based on these studies, the algorithm for investigating lesions between 1 and 2 cm in diameter has been changed. Although the recommendations for investigation of screen-detected lesions in liver were developed for use in patients with cirrhosis, they also apply equally well to patients with chronic hepatitis B or C who may not have fully developed cirrhosis. The pretest probability of HCC being present is high in both situations. For nodules detected in an otherwise normal liver, the pretest probability of HCC is much lower and the guidelines do not apply.

Because radiological diagnosis is so crucial, it is essential that imaging should be carried out properly. Protocols for the diagnosis of HCC are established, which vary by the type of equipment used, and define the amount of contrast to be given, the method of administering the agent, the timing of the studies after administration of contrast, and the thickness of the slices to be collected. The physician ordering the tests should also know whether the studies have been conducted under these conditions. It should be noted that these algorithms cannot be infallible. There will be false-negative results on initial radiology studies, but these tumors should be detected on follow-up imaging before the lesion reaches a size where the likelihood of cure is decreased.

Much has been made of the entity of hypovascular HCC. This is a lesion that enhances less than the surrounding liver tissue both on arterial and venous phase imaging, which is only a diagnostic problem for small lesions (defined as

<2 cm in diameter). Pathological study has shown that the reason for the apparent hypovascularity is that the lesions have a dual blood supply [21]. Histologically, unpaired arteries (no bile duct) are present but in small numbers, and there is still a portal blood supply although reduced. As the tumor matures, the lesion acquires the typical features of HCC and the blood supply becomes more arterialized. Dysplastic nodules also may show unpaired arteries and a reduced portal supply. Therefore, a biopsy is required to distinguish dysplastic nodules from HCC. Unfortunately, even with a needle biopsy, the hallmark features that distinguish a high-grade dysplastic nodule (HGDN) from HCC, namely, stromal invasion, may not be easily detected. Larger HCC may also be hypovascular, and these also need biopsy, although the diagnosis will usually be evident without biopsy.

In addition to morphological features that help distinguish high-grade dysplastic nodules (HGDN) from HCC, there are several histological staining characteristics that may be helpful. Markers of HCC versus benign tissue include glypican [3, 22–24], heat shock protein (HSP) 70 [25], and glutamine synthetase [25]. CD34 staining for vascular endothelium is usually more strongly positive in HCC as unpaired arteries are more clearly identified, whereas in benign tissue, the sinusoidal epithelium stains only weakly. Cytokeratin stains for biliary epithelium (CK7 and CK19) should be negative, and a positive biliary cytokeratin stain makes HCC less likely [26]. Because of the difficulty to make a positive diagnosis in tissue from small lesions, it was recommended that pathologists use the full panel of stains listed above to help distinguish HGDN from HCC. Although occasionally other neoplastic lesions may stain positively with these markers, there should be little difficulty to distinguish these from HCC on morphological grounds.

Thus, the current AASLD recommendations for the diagnosis of HCC are depicted in Fig. 1.1. For lesions smaller than 1 cm, the recommendations remain unchanged. No detailed investigation is required, as most of these will be cirrhotic nodules rather than HCC. However, close follow-up at 3-month intervals is recommended using the technique that first documented the presence of the nodules. If these were detected by screening on ultrasound, then ultrasound is recommended to be the technique of follow-up. Either dynamic MRI or multidetector CT scanner should be used for lesions above 1 cm in

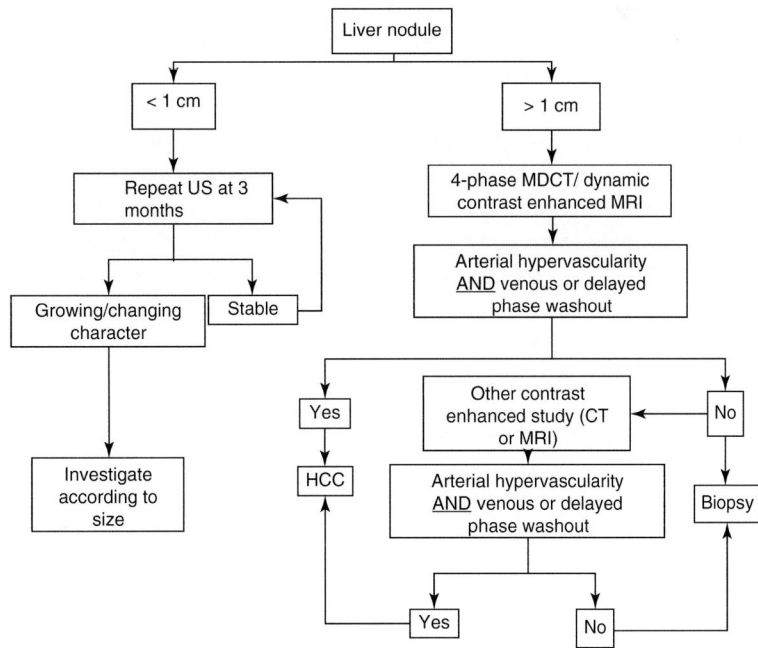

**Fig. 1.1** AASLD diagnostic algorithm. Reprint from Bruix J, Sherman M; American Association for the Study of Liver Diseases. Management of hepatocellular carcinoma: an update. Hepatology. 2011 Mar;53(3):1020–2

diameter. However, contrast-enhanced ultrasound is less specific. If the appearances are typical for HCC on either MRI or CT scan, then no further investigation is required and the diagnosis of HCC is confirmed. If the appearances are not typical for HCC, then one of two strategies is possible. A second contrast-enhanced cross-sectional scan (the other of CT scan or MRI) could be performed. If typical, the diagnosis is confirmed. Alternatively, an atypical study could trigger a biopsy. For this algorithm to be effective, there must be strict adherence to imaging protocols [27, 28] and strict application of the rules regarding vascularity and washout. The presence of arterial enhance alone is insufficient, while the presence of venous washout is essential.

## 1.4 Pathological Diagnosis of Dysplasia and Early HCC

One of the consequences of surveillance programs is the identification of smaller HCCs, as well as dysplastic nodules. The smaller the HCC lesion, the more difficult for us to distinguish malignant from benign nodules. This is true both radiologically and histologically. Recently, a distinction has been made between "very early HCC" [29, 30] and "small" or "progressed" HCC [31, 32]. Early HCC, as defined by Japanese pathologists, is generally hypovascular and has ill-defined margins [9]. Thus, it has a somewhat vague outline on ultrasound and may be hypovascular on CT scanning.

Histologically, there are few unpaired arteries, but the cells show varying grades of dysplasia [33]. There may be invasion of the portal space by hepatocytes, but vessel invasion is absent. These lesions have been called "very early HCC" in the Barcelona Clinic Liver Cancer (BCLC) staging scheme [34]. The pathology of these "very early HCC" lesions has been defined in resected specimens, and therefore, the natural history of these lesions is unclear. However, the presence of small foci of typical HCC within them has been noted, suggesting that these lesions are precursors of typical HCC lesions [29, 31,

32]. The frequency with which these lesions develop typical HCC is unknown either. In contrast, "small" or "progressed" HCC has well-defined margins on ultrasound and exhibits the typical features of well-differentiated HCC on CT and on histology [29, 31, 33]. These lesions often show microvascular invasion, despite their small size [33]. The presence of microvascular invasion suggests that the prognosis of these lesions is less good than for "early HCC" where vascular invasion is rare. However, this has not been proven in clinical studies.

The classification and description of dysplastic nodules and early HCC have been recently revised to harmonize the approaches taken by Western and Japanese pathologists [31]. These studies have been carried out on resected tissue, whereas samples from lesions detected on surveillance usually only have a needle biopsy to evaluate. It is important to understand that rather than being individual discrete states, there is a continuum between HGDN and HCC. This complicates the evaluation of biopsies from small nodules. Patients with liver nodules having a nonspecific vascular profile and negative biopsy should continue to undergo enhanced follow-up as well. There are no data to establish the best follow-up policy so far, but repeated biopsy or follow-up CT/MRI to detect further growth should be considered. There are emerging data indicating that the smaller the lesion, the less likely there is to be microscopic vascular invasion [9].

In addition, smaller lesions are more likely to be associated with treatment that will be curative [30, 35, 36]. Finally, decision analysis also confirms that ideally, for the best outcome, the lesion should be smaller than 2 cm at diagnosis [37]. However, it is equally important not to apply invasive treatment to lesions that do not have any malignant potential and may still regress. This is a fine distinction that is not always possible to make. Another concern about thin needle liver biopsy is the risk of bleeding and needle track seeding. Most studies that report needle track seeding do not specify the lesion size being biopsied [38]. Although the rate of needle track seeding after biopsy of small lesions (<2 cm) has not been accurately measured, it is probably uncommon. The current rate of bleeding from thin needle biopsy of small HCC has not been reported but is probably no different than for biopsy of the liver in general [38, 39].

## 1.5  Diagnostic Recommendations in AASLD Guideline

1. Nodules smaller than 1 cm should be followed with ultrasound at intervals from 3 to 6 months. If there has been no growth over a period of up to 2 years, one can revert to routine surveillance.
2. Nodules larger than 1 cm found on a cirrhotic liver should be investigated further with either four-phase multidetector CT scan or dynamic contrast-enhanced MRI. If the appearances are typical of HCC (i.e., hypervascular in the arterial phase with washout in the portal venous or delayed phase), the lesion should be treated as HCC. If the findings are not characteristic or the vascular profile is not typical, a second contrast-enhanced study with the other imaging modality should be performed, or the lesion should be biopsied.
3. Biopsies of small lesions should be evaluated by expert pathologists. Tissue that is not clearly HCC should be stained with all the

available markers including CD34, CK7, glypican 3, HSP-70, and glutamine synthetase to improve diagnostic accuracy.

4. If the biopsy is negative for patients with HCC, the lesion should be followed by imaging at 3–6 monthly intervals until the nodule either disappears, enlarges, or displays diagnostic characteristics of HCC. If the lesion enlarges but remains atypical for HCC, a repeat biopsy is recommended.

## 1.6  EASL Guidelines

The European Association for the Study of the Liver expert panel proposed the following surveillance recall and diagnostic strategy (Fig. 1.2) [40]. In nodules smaller than 1 cm, which are malignant in less than 50 % of cases, reliable HCC diagnosis is difficult. Thus, close follow-up is recommended. In nodules of 1–2 cm, HCC diagnosis requires positive cytohistology. However, there is a 30–40 % false-negative rate with fine-needle biopsy [41]. A negative result does not rule out malignant disease. Noninvasive diagnostic criteria to be applied solely in patients with cirrhosis and tumors larger than 2 cm were proposed. HCC diagnosis is established by the concomitant finding of two imaging techniques, showing a nodule larger than 2 cm with arterial

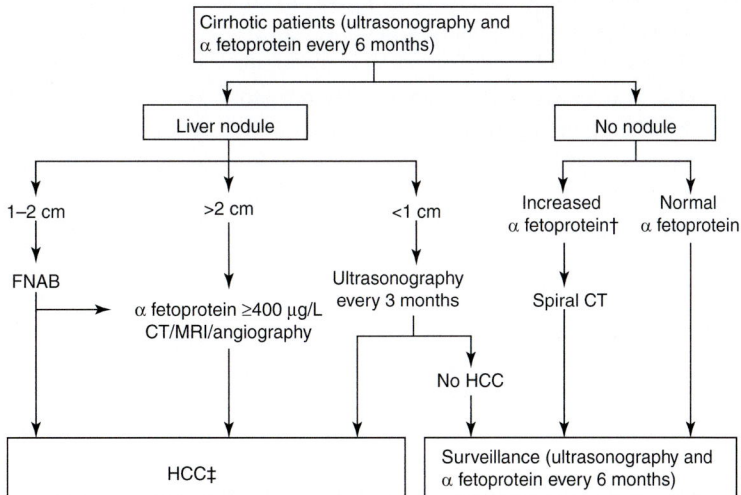

**Fig. 1.2** EASL diagnostic algorithm

hypervascularization, or by one positive imaging technique, showing hypervascularization associated with alpha-fetoprotein concentration higher than 400 ug/L [27]. The accuracy of imaging techniques is rapidly evolving. Ultrasonography plays a key part in the detection of HCC, but its sensitivity to detect additional small nodules is low [42]. New contrast agents might increase the accuracy of this technique and might be relevant to assess treatment response [43]. The best techniques are helical CT and MRI with contrast enhancement, which have an accuracy exceeding 80 % [44]. CT and MRI sensitivity decreases when assessing the extent of the disease. In a comparison of CT and MRI with pathological examination of explanted livers, MRI angiography was more precise in detecting nodules of 1–2 cm than CT scan [12]. However, 20–30 % of intrahepatic tumors, especially those smaller than 10 mm, are not diagnosed preoperatively with any technique. Preliminary data with positron emission tomography are not encouraging for detection of small nodules.

## 1.7 NCCN Guidelines

### 1.7.1 Imaging

Recommendations for imaging in the NCCN Guidelines, if clinical suspicion for HCC is high (e.g., following identification of a liver nodule on ultrasound or in the setting of a rising AFP level), are adapted from the updated guidelines developed by the AASLD [2]. The recommendations included in the NCCN Guidelines apply only to nodules identified in patients with liver cirrhosis. In patients without liver cirrhosis or known liver disease, biopsy should be strongly considered to confirm the diagnosis of HCC.

For patients with an incidental liver mass or nodule found on ultrasound, the guidelines recommend evaluation using one or more of the imaging modalities (at least a three-phase contrast-enhanced CT or MRI including the arterial and portal venous phase) to determine the perfusion characteristics, extent and the number of lesions, vascular anatomy, and extrahepatic disease. The number and type of imaging are dependent on the size of the liver mass or nodule.

Liver lesions <1 cm should be evaluated by at least a three-phase contrast-enhanced CT or MRI or contrast-enhanced ultrasound (CEUS) every 3–6 months, with enlarging lesions evaluated according to size. Patients with lesions stable in size should be followed with imaging every 3–6 months for 2 years (using the same imaging modality that was first used to identify the nodules) then returning to baseline surveillance schedule after 2 years of stability.

Liver nodules greater than 1 cm in size should first be evaluated with three-phase contrast-enhanced CT or MRI. Additional imaging is dependent on the pattern of classic enhancement observed. A finding of two classic enhancements is considered to be diagnostic of HCC, whereas a second imaging (the other CT or MRI) is recommended if there is only one or no classic enhancement pattern. If there are two classic enhancements following additional imaging, the diagnosis of HCC is confirmed. Additional confirmation through tissue sampling (core biopsy is preferred) is recommended if there is only one or no enhancement pattern for patients with liver nodules that are between 1 and 2 cm or greater than 2 cm. For patients with liver nodules between 1 and 2 cm, the NCCN Guidelines have included repeat three-phase imaging in 3 months as an alternative to core biopsy, if there is only one or no classic enhancement pattern following additional imaging.

### 1.7.2 Biopsy

A diagnosis of HCC can be noninvasive in that the biopsy confirmation may not be required. For example, liver nodules greater than 1 cm in size, the finding of two classic enhancement on either one of the recommended imaging modalities (three-phase contrast-enhanced CT or MRI) is sufficient to confirm the diagnosis of HCC. However, a core needle biopsy (preferred) or a fine-needle aspiration biopsy (FNAB) is recommended when zero or one classic arterial enhancement is observed by the recommended imaging method [18].

Nevertheless, the use of biopsy to diagnose HCC is limited by several factors including sampling error, particularly when lesions are less than 1 cm [2, 45]. Patients for whom a nondiagnostic biopsy result is obtained should be followed closely, and subsequent additional imaging and/or biopsy is recommended if a change in nodule size is observed. The guidelines emphasize that a growing mass with a negative biopsy does not rule out HCC. Continual monitoring with a multidisciplinary review including surgeons is recommended.

### 1.7.3 Serum Biomarkers

Although serum AFP has long been used as a marker for HCC, it is not a sensitive or specific diagnostic test for HCC. Serum AFP levels >400 ng/ml are observed only in small percentage of patients with HCC. In a series of 1158 patients with HCC, only 18 % of patients had values >400 ng/ml [46]. In patients with chronic liver disease, an elevated AFP could be more indicative of HCC in non-infected patients [47]. Furthermore, AFP can also be elevated in intrahepatic cholangiocarcinoma and some metastases from colorectal cancer [2]. AFP testing can be useful when combined with other test results to guide the management of patients for whom a diagnosis of HCC is suspected. An elevated AFP level in conjunction with imaging results showing the presence of a larger liver mass has been shown to have a high positive predictive value for HCC in two retrospective studies involving small number of patients [10, 48].

The updated AASLD guidelines no longer recommend AFP testing as part of diagnostic evaluation [4]. The panel considers an imaging finding of classic enhancement to be more definitive in this setting since the level of serum AFP may be elevated in those with certain nonmalignant conditions, as well as within normal limits in a substantial percentage of patients with HCC [49], which is in agreement with the updated AASLD guidelines recommendation. Four additional imaging studies (CT or MRI) are recommended for patients with a rising serum AFP level in the absence of a liver mass. If no liver mass is detected following measurement of an elevated AFP level, the patient should be followed with AFP testing and liver imaging every 3 months.

Other serum biomarkers being studied in this setting include des-gamma-carboxy prothrombin (DCP), also known as protein induced by vitamin K absence-II (PIVKA-II), and lens culinaris agglutinin-reactive AFP (AFP-L3), an isoform of AFP [15, 50–52]. Although AFP was found to be more sensitive than DCP or AFP-L3 in detecting early-stage and very early-stage HCC in a recent retrospective case-control study, none of these biomarkers were considered optimal in this setting [47]. A recent case-control study involving patients with hepatitis C enrolled in the large, randomized HALT-C trial who developed HCC showed that a combination of AFP and DCP is superior to either biomarker alone as a complimentary assay to screening [53].

## References

1. WHO. Globocan 2008. http://globocan.iarc.fr. n.d. [Cited 19 Oct 2013].
2. Bruix J, Sherman M. American Association for the Study of Liver Diseases. Management of hepatocellular carcinoma: an update. Hepatology. 2011;53:1020–2.
3. Benson 3rd AB, Abrams TA, Ben-Josef E, et al. NCCN clinical practice guidelines in oncology: hepatobiliary cancers. J Natl Compr Canc Netw. 2009;7:350–91.
4. Llovet JM, Ducreux M, Lencioni R, Di Bisceglie AM, Galle PR, Dufour JF, Greten TF, et al. European Association for Study of Liver; European Organisation for Research and Treatment of Cancer. EASL-EORTC clinical practice guidelines: management of hepatocellular carcinoma. Eur J Cancer. 2012;48:599–641.
5. Sato Y, Sekine T, Ohwada S. Alpha-fetoprotein-producing rectal cancer: calculated tumor marker doubling time. J Surg Oncol. 1994;55:265–8.
6. Adachi Y, Tsuchihashi J, Shiraishi N, Yasuda K, Etoh T, Kitano S. AFP-producing gastric carcinoma: multivariate analysis of prognostic factors in 270 patients. Oncology. 2003;65:95–101.
7. Forns X, Ampurdanes S, Llovet JM, Aponte J, Quinto L, Martinez-Bauer E, Bruguera M, et al. Identification of chronic hepatitis C patients without hepatic fibrosis by a simple predictive model. Hepatology. 2002;36:986–92.
8. Moriyama M, Matsumura H, Aoki H, Shimizu T, Nakai K, Saito T, Yamagami H, et al. Long-term outcome, with monitoring of platelet counts, in patients with

chronic hepatitis C and liver cirrhosis after interferon therapy. Intervirology. 2003;46:296–307.

9. Kojiro M. Focus on dysplastic nodules and early hepatocellular carcinoma: an eastern point of view. Liver Transpl. 2004;10:S3–8.

10. Levy I, Greig PD, Gallinger S, Langer B, Sherman M. Resection of hepatocellular carcinoma without preoperative tumor biopsy. Ann Surg. 2001;234:206–9. Hepatology, Vol. 000, No. 000, 2010 Bruix and Sherman 29.

11. Torzilli G, Makuuchi M, Inoue K, Takayama T, Sakamoto Y, Sugawara Y, Kubota K, et al. No-mortality liver resection for hepatocellular carcinoma in cirrhotic and noncirrhotic patients: is there a way? A prospective analysis of our approach. Arch Surg. 1999;134:984–92.

12. Burrel M, Llovet JM, Ayuso C, Iglesias C, Sala M, Miquel R, Caralt T, et al. MRI angiography is superior to helical CT for detection of HCC prior to liver transplantation: an explant correlation. Hepatology. 2003;38:1034–42.

13. Yu JS, Kim KW, Kim EK, Lee JT, Yoo HS. Contrast enhancement of small hepatocellular carcinoma: usefulness of three successive early image acquisitions during multiphase dynamic MR imaging. AJR Am J Roentgenol. 1999;173:597–604.

14. Mueller GC, Hussain HK, Carlos RC, Nghiem HV, Francis IR. Effectiveness of MR imaging in characterizing small hepatic lesions: routine versus expert interpretation. AJR Am J Roentgenol. 2003;180:673–80.

15. Forner A, Vilana R, Ayuso C, Bianchi L, Sole M, Ayuso JR, Boix L, et al. Diagnosis of hepatic nodules 20 mm or smaller in cirrhosis: prospective validation of the noninvasive diagnostic criteria for hepatocellular carcinoma. Hepatology. 2008;47:97–104.

16. Leoni S, Piscaglia F, Golfieri R, Camaggi V, Vidili G, Pini P, Bolondi L. The impact of vascular and nonvascular findings on the noninvasive diagnosis of small hepatocellular carcinoma based on the EASL and AASLD criteria. Am J Gastroenterol. 2010;105:599–609.

17. Khalili KKT, Jang HJ, Haider MA, Guindi M, Sherman M. Implementation of AASLD hepatocellular carcinoma practice guideline in North America: two years of experience. Hepatology. 2008;48:362A.

18. Sangiovanni A, Manini MA, Iavarone M, Romeo R, Forzenigo LV, Fraquelli M, Massironi S, et al. The diagnostic and economic impact of contrast imaging technique in the diagnosis of small hepatocellular carcinoma in cirrhosis. Gut. 2010;59:570–1.

19. Rimola J, Forner A, Reig M, Vilana R, de Lope CR, Ayuso C, Bruix J. Cholangiocarcinoma in cirrhosis: absence of contrast washout in delayed phases by magnetic resonance imaging avoids misdiagnosis of hepatocellular carcinoma. Hepatology. 2009;50:791–8.

20. Vilana R, Forner A, Bianchi L, Garcia-Criado A, Rimola J, Rodrı´guez de Lope C. Intrahepatic peripheral cholangiocarcinoma in cirrhosis patients may display a vascular pattern similar to hepatocellular carcinoma on contrast-enhanced ultrasound. Hepatology. 2010;51:2020–9.

21. Nakashima Y, Nakashima O, Hsia CC, Kojiro M, Tabor E. Vascularization of small hepatocellular carcinomas: correlation with differentiation. Liver. 1999;19:12–8.

22. Kandil D, Leiman G, Allegretta M, Trotman W, Pantanowitz L, Goulart R, Evans M. Glypican-3 immunocytochemistry in liver fine-needle aspirates: a novel stain to assist in the differentiation of benign and malignant liver lesions. Cancer. 2007;111:316–22.

23. Libbrecht L, Bielen D, Verslype C, Vanbeckevoort D, Pirenne J, Nevens F, Desmet V, et al. Focal lesions in cirrhotic explant livers: pathological evaluation and accuracy of pretransplantation imaging examinations. Liver Transpl. 2002;8:749–61.

24. Wang XY, Degos F, Dubois S, Tessiore S, Allegretta M, Guttmann RD, Jothy S, et al. Glypican-3 expression in hepatocellular tumors: diagnostic value for preneoplastic lesions and hepatocellular carcinomas. Hum Pathol. 2006;37:1435–41.

25. Di Tommaso L, Franchi G, Park YN, Fiamengo B, Destro A, Morenghi E, Montorsi M, et al. Diagnostic value of HSP70, glypican 3, and glutamine synthetase in hepatocellular nodules in cirrhosis. Hepatology. 2007;45:725–34.

26. Park YN, Kojiro M, Di Tommaso L, Dhillon AP, Kondo F, Nakano M, Sakamoto M, et al. Ductular reaction is helpful in defining early stromal invasion, small hepatocellular carcinomas, and dysplastic nodules. Cancer. 2007;109:915–23.

27. Lencioni RLJ. Modified recist (mRECIST) assessment for hepatocellular carcinoma. Semin Liver Dis. 2010;30:52–60.

28. Pomfret E, Washburn K, Wald C, Nalesnik M, Douglas D, Russo M, Roberts JP, et al. Report of a national conference on liver allocation in patients with hepatocellular carcinoma in the United States. Liver Transpl. 2010;16:262–78.

29. Sakamoto M, Hirohashi S. Natural history and prognosis of adenomatous hyperplasia and early hepatocellular carcinoma: multi-institutional analysis of 53 nodules followed up for more than 6 months and 141 patients with single early hepatocellular carcinoma treated by surgical resection or percutaneous ethanol injection. Jpn J Clin Oncol. 1998;28:604–8.

30. Takayama T, Makuuchi M, Hirohashi S, Sakamoto M, Yamamoto J, Shimada K, Kosuge T, et al. Early hepatocellular carcinoma as an entity with a high rate of surgical cure. Hepatology. 1998;28:1241–6.

31. Kojiro M, Wanless IR, Alves V, Badve S, Balabaud C, Bedossa P, Bhathal P, et al. The International Consensus Group for Hepatocellular Neoplasia. Pathologic diagnosis of early hepatocellular carcinoma: a report of the international consensus group for hepatocellular neoplasia. Hepatology. 2009;49:658–64.

32. Takayama T, Makuuchi M, Hirohashi S, Sakamoto M, Okazaki N, Takayasu K, Kosuge T, et al. Malignant transformation of adenomatous hyperplasia to hepatocellular carcinoma. Lancet. 1990;336:1150–3.

33. Nakashima Y, Nakashima O, Tanaka M, Okuda K, Nakashima M, Kojiro M. Portal vein invasion and intrahepatic micrometastasis in small hepatocellular carcinoma by gross type. Hepatol Res. 2003;26:142–7.

34. Forner ARM, Rodrigruez de Lope C, Bruix J. Current strategy for staging and treatment: the BCLC update and future prospects. Semin Liver Dis. 2010;30:61–74.

35. Sala M, Llovet JM, Vilana R, Bianchi L, Sole M, Ayuso C, Bru C, et al. Initial response to percutaneous ablation predicts survival in patients with hepatocellular carcinoma. Hepatology. 2004;40:1352–60.

36. Vilana R, Bruix J, Bru C, Ayuso C, Sole M, Rodes J. Tumor size determines the efficacy of percutaneous ethanol injection for the treatment of small hepatocellular carcinoma. Hepatology. 1992;16:353–7.

37. Bremner KE, Bayoumi AM, Sherman M, Krahn MD. Management of solitary 1 cm to 2 cm liver nodules in patients with compensated cirrhosis: a decision analysis. Can J Gastroenterol. 2007;21:491–500.

38. Silva MA, Hegab B, Hyde C, Guo B, Buckels JA, Mirza DF. Needle track seeding following biopsy of liver lesions in the diagnosis of hepatocellular cancer: a systematic review and meta-analysis. Gut. 2008;57:1592–6.

39. Stigliano R, Marelli L, Yu D, Davies N, Patch D, Burroughs AK. Seeding following percutaneous diagnostic and therapeutic approaches for hepatocellular carcinoma. What is the risk and the outcome? Seeding risk for percutaneous approach of HCC. Cancer Treat Rev. 2007;33:437–47.

40. Bruix J, Sherman M, Llovet JM, et al. Clinical management of hepatocellular carcinoma: conclusions of the Barcelona-2000 EASL Conference. J Hepatol. 2001;35:421–30.

41. Durand F, Regimbeau JM, Belghiti J, et al. Assessment of the benefits and risks of percutaneous biopsy before surgical resection of hepatocellular carcinoma. J Hepatol. 2001;35:254–8.

42. Kim CK, Lim JH, Lee WJ. Detection of hepatocellular carcinomas and dysplastic nodules in cirrhotic liver: accuracy of ultrasonography in transplant patients. J Ultrasound Med. 2001;20:99–104.

43. Lencioni R, Cioni D, Bartolozzi C. Tissue harmonic and contrastspecific imaging: back to gray scale ultrasound. Eur Radiol. 2002;12:151–65.

44. Choi D, Kim SH, Lim JH, et al. Detection of hepatocellular carcinoma: combined T2-weighted and dynamic gadoliniumenhanced MRI versus combined CT during arterial portography and CT hepatic arteriography. J Comput Assist Tomogr. 2001;25:777–85.

45. Volk ML, Marrero JA. Early detection of liver cancer: diagnosis and management. Curr Gastroenterol Rep. 2008;10:60–6.

46. Farinati F, Marino D, De Giorgio M, et al. Diagnositc and prognostic role of alpha-fetoprotein in hepatocellular carcinoma: both or neither? Am J Gastroenterol. 2006;101:524–32.

47. Trevisani F, D'Intino PE, Morselli-Labate AM, et al. Serum alpha-fetoprotein for diagnosis of hepatocellular carcinoma in patients with chronic liver disease: influence of HbsAg and anti-HCV status. J Hepatol. 2001;34:570–5.

48. Torzilli G, Minagawa M, Takayama T, et al. Accurate preoperative evaluation of liver mass lesions without fine-needle biopsy. Hepatology. 1999;30:889–93.

49. Lok AS, Lai CL. Alpha-fetoprotein monitoring in Chinese patients with chronic hepatitis B virus infection: role in the early detection of hepatocellular carcinoma. Hepatology. 1989;9:110–5.

50. Debruyne EN, Delanghe JR. Diagnosing and monitoring hepatocellular carcinoma with alpha-fetoprotein: new aspects and applications. Clin Chim Acta. 2008;395:19–26.

51. Durazo FA, Blatt LM, Corey WG, et al. Des-gamma-carboxyprothrombin, alpha-fetoprotein and AFP-L3 in patients with chronic hepatitis, cirrhosis and hepatocellular carcinoma. J Gastroenterol Hepatol. 2008;23:1541–8.

52. Marrero JA, Feng Z, Wang Y, et al. Alpha-fetoprotein, des-gamma carboxyprothrombin, and lectin-bound alpha-fetoprotein in early hepatocellular carcinoma. Gastroenterology. 2009;137:110–8.

53. Lok AS, Sterling RK, Everhart JE, et al. Des-gamma-carboxyprothrombin and alpha-fetoprotein as biomarkers for the early detection of hepatocellular carcinoma. Gastroenterology. 2010;138:493–502.

# Pathobiologic Characteristics of Small Hepatocellular Carcinoma

Wenming Cong, Xinyuan Lu, and Wanyee Lau

## 2.1 Small HCC Is Not Equivalent to Early HCC

Early diagnosis and treatment of cancer have long been established as basic principles of modern surgical oncology. There is no doubt that a better understanding of the pathobiological features of small hepatocellular carcinoma (SHCC) will provide clinicians with the pathobiological basis to better treat these tumors and to improve long-term survivals of patients. For relatively small HCC, several designations such as "early HCC" and "subclinical HCC" [1] have been proposed. The definitions of these tumors are based mainly upon tumor size, and each definition uses a different size. The concept of SHCC can be traced back to the late 1970s [2, 3], when SHCC was considered as the most significant prognostic factor of long-term survival.

However, no consensus has been reached among researchers or clinicians who designed clinical practice guidelines which have been accepted worldwide on the size criterion for SHCC. As a consequence, a confusing plethora of size standards to define SHCC, including 5 cm [2–4], 4.5 cm [5], 4 cm [6], 3.5 cm [7], 3 cm [8–11], 2.5 cm [12], and 2 cm [13–16] has been used.

According to the database of the Department of Pathology at the Eastern Hepatobiliary Surgery Hospital (EHBH), Shanghai, China, the largest special hepatic surgical hospital in China, 2459 and 3092 liver resections for HCCs were carried out in the years 2007 and 2011, respectively. The resected specimens showed HCCs with a diameter of $\leq 2$ cm and $\leq 3$ cm to account for 9.3 % and 19 %, and 10.3 % and 31.4 %, respectively. These figures were obviously higher than the 2.6 % and 8.7 % reported before 1997 [17]. With the exception of micro or minute HCCs ($\leq 1$ cm), which corresponded to carcinoma in situ or very early HCC, our previous studies on pathobiological features of solitary HCCs showed that by dividing HCC into subgroups of 1-cm-diameter increments, there were no significant differences in the clinicopathological features among the subgroups of HCCs, which ranged from 1 to 3 cm (SHCC) or among the subgroups of large HCCs (LHCCs), which ranged over 3 cm. However, if 3 cm was used as a cutoff for SHCC, significant differences were observed between the groups of SHCC and LHCC ($P < 0.05$–0.01) [18]. These differences included histological grades I–II versus III–IV, the presence or absence of capsular invasion/portal venous tumor thrombi/satellite nodules, invasive growth patterns, and overall survival and recurrence-free survival. Multivariate Cox regression

W. Cong, MD, PhD (✉) • X. Lu, MD
Department of Pathology, Eastern Hepatobiliary Surgery Hospital, Second Military Medical University, Shanghai, China
e-mail: wmcong@gmail.com

W. Lau, MD, DSc, FACS, FRCS, FRACS(Hon)
The Chinese University of Hong Kong, Shatin, New Territories, Hong Kong SAR, China

© Springer Science+Business Media Dordrecht 2016
M. Chen et al. (eds.), *Radiofrequency Ablation for Small Hepatocellular Carcinoma*,
DOI 10.1007/978-94-017-7258-7_2

analyses showed that tumor size ≤3 cm was an independent prognostic factor of overall and recurrence-free survivals [18, 19]. Similar results were also reported by Pawlik et al. [20].

An early HCC, in general, is a tumor at an early developmental stage characterized by well-differentiation on histology, with noninvasive growth pattern and a more favorable long-term prognosis after curative treatment. The Liver Cancer Study Group of Japan defined early HCC as a well-differentiated HCC with an obscure tumor margin [21]. Early HCC is often detected in cirrhotic livers, and it shows as a hypovascular nodule in the arterial phase of an intravenous contrast enhanced computed tomographic (CT) scan [22].

Although tumor size has been proposed as a criterion to define early HCC, there is still no consensus on the size that should be used. Mazzaferro et al. [23] defined early-stage HCC for transplantation to be a single tumor <5 cm or two to three tumors all <3 cm, with no evidence of extrahepatic tumor (the Milan criteria). Nathan et al. [24] defined early HCC as tumors ≤5 cm and without metastatic disease, nodal metastasis, extrahepatic extension, or major vascular invasion. In the early study of the Barcelona Clinic Liver Cancer (BCLC) group, early HCC was defined as a single tumor ≤5 cm [25, 26]. However, in the recent BCLC classification, very early HCC is defined as well-differentiated tumors ≤2 cm in diameter without any vascular invasion or satellites, and early HCC is defined as HCC ≤2 cm with microscopic vascular invasion/satellites, or 2–5-cm well-differentiated/moderately differentiated HCC without any vascular invasion/satellites, or two or three well-differentiated nodules <3 cm [27, 28]. However, the BCLC group reported that nearly 60 % of their SHCCs, which were less than 2 cm, had moderate to poor differentiation [15], whereas Sakamoto and Hirohashi [29] defined early HCC as a well-differentiated HCC (Edmondson's grade I or grade I with a minor component of grade II), negative for tumor staining on angiographic examination, and regardless of tumor size.

While small HCC is usually defined on tumor size, early HCC is still commonly defined on histopathological grounds. It should be emphasized that a small HCC is not always necessarily equivalent to an early HCC as defined histologically, although most early HCCs are less than 2 cm in its greatest diameter [30]. In the Italian Liver Cancer group (ITA.LI.-CA)'s classification, an early HCC is defined as a solitary HCC smaller than 5 cm because SHCC below 2 cm is rare [16]. In the current revised version of the BCLC system, as released by the American Association for the Study of Liver Diseases, patients diagnosed at an early stage are defined as having single or three nodules below 3 cm each [31, 32]. On the other hand, other scholars defined pathologically early HCC to correspond to carcinoma in situ [33] and clinically early HCC is characterized by a locally curable tumor, which has a favorable long-term survival outcome [34].

Early HCC with its benign behavior is at an early phase in the progression of HCC, while small HCC may already have developed malignant behavior. Although a small HCC is not equivalent to an early "benign" tumor because some aggressive HCC can metastasize when it is still small in size, most researchers agree that with increase in size of a small HCC, there is a gradual change in pathobiological behavior of the tumor. Tumor size has been shown to be the best predictor of tumor behavior [35].

Conceptually, the criteria used to define SHCC are tumor size-based while early HCC are biological behavior-based. A small-size HCC does not absolutely mean a tumor having early biological behavior. Although pathologically, SHCC ≤ 3 cm tends to show relatively benign behavior, a small proportion of SHCC presents with aneuploid DNA content [8, 36, 37] and harbors microvascular invasion [38, 39]. These more malignant features happen even in a minute HCC 0.6 cm in diameter, [18]. As a consequence, SHCC can further be divided into two clinicopathological subtypes: early SHCC and progressive SHCC. In patients with a single tumor, tumor size has no impact on survival in patients with no vascular invasion or microvascular invasion, irrespective of how the tumor size was dichotomized [14]. In HCC ≤ 2 cm, patients who have suspicious features of gross invasive type of tumors on preoperative imaging are at a high risk of having pathological microinvasion. In such patients, hepatic resection with a wide tumor margin is recommended. Even a SHCC $\leq 3$ cm should be surgically resected with reasonable margins. As approximately 80 % of vascular invasion or micrometastatic foci are located within 1 cm of the primary SHCC, it is important to resect or to ablate the tumor with an adequate width of surrounding tissues (of > 1 cm) to prevent recurrence coming from residual tumor cells. Therefore, no matter what therapeutic options are chosen for SHCC, curative treatment with adequate safety margins should always be given.

## 2.2 Pathobiological Characteristics of SHCC

Like many other human solid tumors which undergo initiation, promotion, and progression, HCC possesses a similar multi-stage evolution model in its hepatocarcinogenesis [40–42]. In general, the smaller the tumor, the greater is the chance of radical cure and the longer is the postoperative long-term survival. On the other hand, the more advanced the lesion, the lower is the likelihood that therapy is curative. Also, the smaller the lesion, the closer it lies to the dysplasia/neoplasia boundary, the more difficult it is to be certain on histological analysis whether the lesion is malignant (Edmondson and Steiner's grade I). We herein briefly review the history in the study of SHCC, analyze the advantages and limitations of using different criteria to define SHCC, and discuss the pathobiological characteristics of SHCC and their clinical significance.

### 2.2.1 The Features of a SHCC $\leq 5$ cm

In the mid to late 1970s, Chinese surgeons Dr. Tang ZY et al. [2] and Dr. Wu MC et al. [3] first put forward the concept of SHCC. This has a milestone-like significance to give basic scientists and clinical researchers to direct their research from large HCC (LHCC) at the middle-advanced stage to SHCC at the early developmental stage. At that time, a HCC $\leq 5$ cm in diameter was defined as SHCC based on the clinical information that about 70 % of HCC patients

who were subclinical (without any symptoms) harbored a tumor $\leq 5$ cm in diameter. In contrast, about 70 % of subjects harboring a tumor > 5 cm showed obvious clinical symptoms. Patients with a tumor measuring $\leq 5$ cm in diameter survived longer than those with tumors > 5 cm in diameter [2, 3]. Since then, this concept that patients who have an early-stage HCC are those who present with an asymptomatic single HCC $\leq 5$ cm has been widely accepted even up to now [14, 20, 24, 25, 43–46]. Also, the AJCC/UICC seventh edition of TNM classification uses a cutoff tumor size of 5 cm in the T3a HCC staging [47].

With advances in radiographic diagnostic techniques, much smaller liver tumors can now be detected. As more studies show improvement in long-term prognosis with treatment of solitary HCCs smaller than 5 cm, using 5 cm as the SHCC criterion in modern hepatic surgery seems too large when compared with the concept of small tumors of other organs [48–51].

### 2.2.2 The Features of a SHCC $\leq 3$ cm

In 1981, the Liver Cancer Pathological Study Group of China proposed a macroscopic classification of HCC, and HCC $\leq 3$ cm in diameter was classified as an independent type [52]. In 1986, Ebara et al. [53] reported on 22 Japanese patients with minute HCC of less than 3 cm in diameter who received no special treatment. The serum alpha-fetoprotein levels in these patients were low, and they were rarely useful for diagnosis. However, this tumor marker level tended to increase when the mass had attained a diameter greater than 3 cm. In the following year, the Japanese pathologists proposed a gross classification of five subtypes for SHCC $\leq 3$ cm in diameter [54].

We started to compare the relationship between HCC size and DNA ploidy in 1988 to better understand the pathobiological features of SHCC in its early stage [36]. The results showed the majority of HCCs $\leq 3$ cm in diameter maintained DNA diploidy. These tumors were characterized by relatively "benign" behaviors, which included a clear tumor margin with or without a complete fibrous capsule, well cell differentiation, almost no satellites and microvascular invasion, and they were easy to be radically resected resulting in long-term postoperative survival [8, 19, 55]. In comparison, HCCs > 3 cm in diameter mainly showed DNA aneuploidy with obvious malignant behaviors, which included poor cell differentiation, capsular invasion, a high-frequency of satellite nodules and tumor thrombus formation, and a high-risk of residual tumor after radical treatment with relatively poor survival outcomes [8, 19, 55]. As a consequence, we proposed that HCC approaching 3 cm in diameter is reaching an important turning point for critical transformation, with a change from relatively "benign" behaviors to a more aggressive progression. The 3-cm cutoff seems to be the most suitable point to define SHCC [8, 36].

In 1994, Ng et al. [37] reported that DNA ploidy may supplement other predictors in prognostication when HCCs are stratified into small and large tumors at a cutoff point of 5 cm in diameter. Interestingly, a recent study on 12 methylation genes showed that all CpG positions in APC, GSTP1, and CFTR were more highly methylated in small HCCs less than 3 cm than in non-tumorous liver tissues ($p < 0.05$), and RASSF1A, CCND2, and APC were frequently positive (91–100 % of cases examined) in well-differentiated HCCs, small HCCs less than 3 cm, and Stages I and II HCCs [56]. Notably, the three-marker combination of RASSF1A, CCND2, and SPINT2 demonstrated the highest sensitivity and accuracy (89–95 % and 89–97 %), respectively, for all HCCs and early HCCs, and they correctly diagnosed all HCC cases in the early HCC group [56]. Likewise, Llovet et al. [27] found the expressions of GPC3, survivin, and LYVE1 to be significantly increased in dysplastic nodules, early HCC (mean size, 2 ± 0.6 cm, range, 0.9–3 cm) and advanced HCC, and the diagnostic accuracy of this three-gene set was 94 %. These studies suggest that there is a relevant molecular basis for SHCC in its early progression stage.

Histopathologically, when HCCs grow to over 2–3 cm in diameter, the well-differentiated cancerous tissues are completely replaced by moderately differentiated cancer tissues, and it is uncommon to see well-differentiated cancer tissues in tumors larger than 3 cm in diameter [57]. Tumor size larger than 3 cm is also a main risk factor of local recurrence [58], and a wider resection margin is recommended for HCCs more than 3 cm than those less than 3 cm to eradicate all micrometastases aiming to achieve good long-term survivals [59].

Many multi-center studies have reported that the postoperative survival of patients with SHCCs ≤ 3 cm in diameter was significantly better than that of patients with LHCCs > 3 cm in diameter [60–66]. Therefore, a HCC ≤ 3 cm in diameter was named as an SHCC in the first edition of the Barcelona Clinic Liver Cancer (BCLC) staging system in 1999 [4] and in the HCC staging system proposed by the Chinese Society of Liver Cancer in 2001 [67], and it was kept in the 2011 edition (http://www.moh.gov.cn). Also, a consensus-based treatment algorithm for HCC proposed by the Japan Society of Hepatology (JSH), which was revised in 2010 [68], set the cutoff point at ≤ 3 cm.

A 3 cm tumor can be completely ablated with a 10-min application of percutaneous radiofrequency ablation [69], and percutaneous ethanol injection prolongs patient survival with survival rates similar to surgical resection, especially for tumors < 3 cm [70, 71]. Therefore, it is important to diagnose and treat HCC < 3 cm.

### 2.2.3 The Features of a SHCC ≤ 2 cm

In both the fourth edition (1987) [72] and the fifth edition (1997) [73] of the Tumor-Node-Metastasis (TNM) classification for HCC, ≤ 2 cm was used as the size criterion for T1 HCC as proposed by AJCC/UICC. This approximates to the size of a lesion that could be detected on screening, and this poses some difficulties in diagnosis. However, many scholars reported that these two versions of the TNM classifications were not of prognostic value [45, 74–76]. In the current seventh edition of the TNM system [47], T1 HCC was re-defined as a tumor of any size but without microvascular invasion. Meanwhile, the Liver Cancer Study Group of Japan (LCSGJ) proposed its own TNM staging using a non-strict 2-cm standard [77]. However, this revision was primarily based on data collected from LCSGJ's data, which were collected from more than 800 institutes through a Japanese nationwide survey during a 6–10-year-period [13].

The concept of a very early stage of HCC or carcinoma in situ for a HCC < 2 cm in size for which a definitive diagnosis is often difficult to establish first appeared in the second edition of the BCLC staging system in 2003 [28]. The BCLC staging system has since become widely accepted in clinical practice, and it is also commonly used in clinical trials on new drugs for HCC. Unfortunately, almost all studies on SHCC ≤ 2 cm which have been reported in medical literature are based on small samples [13, 15, 16, 30, 38, 45, 64, 78–87] or without clearly mentioning the actual sample size [31, 68, 88]. Farinati et al. [16], from the Italian Liver Cancer group (ITA.LI.CA) indicated that their patients with the "very early HCC" of smaller than 2 cm were too few (3 %) to perform an internal validation analysis or to make a definition of this disease stage clinically useful. Therefore, they preferred to use 5 cm as the cutoff point. Although review articles on these classifications have been published, none of these classifications have received universal acceptance.

## 2.2.4 Pathological Patterns of SHCC

Nakashima et al. [89] divided small HCC of less than 3 cm in diameter into the vaguely nodular type with indistinct margins, the single nodular type, the single nodular type with extranodular growth, and the confluent multinodular type. None of the vaguely nodular type had intrahepatic metastasis or portal vein invasion. The reason why an early HCC shows a vague (indistinct) nodular pattern remains unclear. We speculate that in the early developing stage of SHCC, patients may lack an effective immune response or defense ability, or patients with SHCC have an early/precirrhotic-stage cirrhosis in the noncancerous tissue, which may lead to the absence of a fibrous capsule in early HCC [19].

Histologically, early SHCC usually shows well differentiation with a thin trabecular pattern and lacks prominent cellular and structural atypia. None of the vaguely nodular type showed intrahepatic metastasis or portal vein invasion. Based on histological grading, Sasaki et al. [90] classified SHCC ≤ 3 cm into early HCC, well-differentiated HCC, and moderately or poorly differentiated HCC. The 5-year survival rates of patients in the above three groups were 100 %, 60%, and 27 %, respectively.

SHCC of the vaguely nodular type, which is one of the subtypes derived from the gross classification of HCC of less than 3 cm in diameter, is considered as a macroscopic characteristic of early-stage HCCs by the LCSGJ [54, 80] and the International Consensus Group for Hepatocellular Neoplasia (ICGHN) [38]. However, many SHCCs of the vaguely nodular type as diagnosed by Japanese pathologists tend to be recognized as high-grade dysplastic nodules (HGDN) by Western pathologists [88, 91]. Although pathologic diagnostic criteria for SHCC have been fully described, which include that the lesions should present with intratumoral portal tracts and stromal invasion [38, 88, 92, 93], it is difficult to identify morphological correlates of malignant behavior at the boundary between premalignant and malignant states, because dysplasia and early neoplasia share many common histological features. Many well-differentiated SHCC and HGDN show similar pathological features, such as vaguely nodular appearances, increased cell density, thin trabecular pattern, and unpaired arteries [94]. Individual discrepancy probably exists among even expert hepatopathologists in the histological diagnosis between HGDN and well-differentiated SHCC with a vaguely nodular appearance. For example, "stromal invasion" is considered the most objective and reliable criterion to distinguish a well-differentiated HCC from a HGDN [95]. However, from our experience based on more than 30,000 archived surgical HCC specimens in the database of the Department of Pathology, EHBH, while intranodular portal tracts seem more likely to appear in dysplastic nodules, stromal invasion into portal tracts or fibrous septa may sometimes but not commonly seen in early SHCC. Any nodule in a cirrhotic liver with a diameter of >3 cm should be regarded as very suspicious of HCC, because benign nodules of this size is rare [96]. Anyway, diagnosis by hepatopathologists on minute nodules remains a challenge, and this has prompted hepatopathologists to develop new diagnostic tools using immunostaining, gene expression assessment, or molecular classification. In conclusion, early diagnosis and definitive treatment are the keys to achieve good long-term survival outcome.

## 2.3　Classification of T Staging of HCC According to Size of HCC, How Small Is Small?

The Tumor-Node-Metastasis (TNM) staging system is one of the most widely accepted system for prediction of prognosis [97, 98]. The American Joint Committee on Cancer (AJCC)/ International Union Against Cancer (UICC) staging system stratifies the prognosis of hepatocellular carcinoma (HCC) patients by using a TNM classification which considers tumor size and number, vascular invasion, lymph node involvement, and extra-hepatic metastasis. The AJCC/UICC has published the seventh edition of the TNM staging system in 2009 [47]. In the TNM staging system, tumor number, vascular invasion, lymph node involvement, and extra-hepatic metastasis are relatively easy to define. However, tumor size in the T staging of HCC changed from 2 cm (AJCC/UICC fifth edition) to 5 cm (AJCC/UICC sixth edition and AJCC/ UICC seventh edition). The reason for the change was "All solitary tumors without vascular invasion, regardless of size, are classified as T1 because of similar prognosis." However, our experience suggests that this change is too radical because it did not consider an HCC of 3 cm. We will review the importance of an HCC of 3 cm on prognosis, biological behavior, and its impact on any therapeutic guideline.

### 2.3.1　Size of HCC on Prognosis

It has been increasingly reported that size of HCC is a prognostic factor. The AJCC first edition cancer staging manual was reported in 1977, the seventh edition was updated in 2009 (Table 2.1). In the first edition, the TNM stage of HCC was not described. In the second edition of the AJCC Cancer Staging system, an early HCC was defined as a tumor size of ≤3 cm. Among the third–fifth editions of the AJCC Cancer Staging system, this tumor size was defined as ≤2 cm.

From the sixth edition of the AJCC Cancer Staging system, the tumor size was defined as ≤5 cm. It was described in the sixth edition that "All solitary tumors without vascular invasion, regardless of size, are classified as T1 because of similar prognosis" [99]. However, our two large cohort studies revealed that the cumulative survival rates were significantly different among groups of patients with HCC ≤2 cm, 3 cm, and 5 cm [8, 18]. In addition, our published data also supported that patients with HCC above or below 3 cm had significantly different survival rates [18]. The updated BCLC also considered HCC of 3 cm to be the main factor in choice of any potentially curative option such as curative liver resection, ablation, or transplantation [100].

### 2.3.2　Size of HCC Versus Pathological Features

Nakashima et al. [89], Sasaki et al. [90], and our data proposed that the prognosis is related to tumor size, pathologic stage, growth pattern, gross feature, histological feature, clinical stage, and biological stage [101].

### 2.3.3　Size of HCC Versus Biological Behavior

Our study proposed that an HCC approaching 3 cm in diameter is reaching an important turning point for critical transformation, which

**Table 2.1** Illustration of TNM stages of HCC

| Edition | Publication year | Effective year | T-stage |
|---|---|---|---|
| 1 | 1977 | 1978 | None |
| 2 | 1983 | 1984 | T1 Small solitary tumor (<3 cm) confined to one lobe |
|  |  |  | T2 Large tumor (>3 cm) confined to one lobe, T2a: single tumor nodule, T2b: multiple tumor nodule (any size) |
|  |  |  | T3 Tumor involving both major lobes, T3a: single tumor nodule (with direct extension), T3b: multiple tumor nodules |
|  |  |  | T4 Tumor invading adjacent organs |
| 3 | 1988 | 1989 | T1 Solitary tumor 2 cm or less in greatest dimension without vascular invasion |
|  |  |  | T2 Solitary tumor 2 cm or less in greatest dimension with vascular invasion, or multiple tumors limited to one lobe, none more than 2 cm in greatest dimension without vascular invasion, or solitary tumor more than 2 cm in greatest dimension without vascular invasion |
|  |  |  | T3 Solitary tumor more than 2 cm in greatest dimension with vascular, or multiple tumors limited to one lobe, none more than 2 cm in greatest dimension, with vascular invasion, or multiple tumors limited to one lobe, any more than 2 cm in greatest dimension, with or without vascular invasion |
|  |  |  | T4 Multiple tumors in more than one lobe, or tumors involving a major branch of portal or hepatic veins |
| 4 | 1992 | 1993 | T1 Solitary tumor 2 cm or less in greatest dimension without vascular invasion |
|  |  |  | T2 Solitary tumor 2 cm or less in greatest dimension with vascular invasion, or multiple tumors limited to one lobe, none more than 2 cm in greatest dimension without vascular invasion, or solitary tumor more than 2 cm in greatest dimension without vascular invasion |
|  |  |  | T3 Solitary tumor more than 2 cm in greatest dimension with vascular, or multiple tumors limited to one lobe, none more than 2 cm in greatest dimension, with vascular invasion, or multiple tumors limited to one lobe, any more than 2 cm in greatest dimension, with or without vascular invasion |
|  |  |  | T4 Multiple tumors in more than one lobe, or tumors involving a major branch of portal or hepatic veins |
| 5 | 1997 | 1998 | T1 Solitary tumor 2 cm or less in greatest dimension without vascular invasion |
|  |  |  | T2 Solitary tumor 2 cm or less in greatest dimension with vascular invasion, or multiple tumors limited to one lobe, none more than 2 cm in greatest dimension without vascular invasion, or solitary tumor more than 2 cm in greatest dimension without vascular invasion |
|  |  |  | T3 Solitary tumor more than 2 cm in greatest dimension with vascular, or multiple tumors limited to one lobe, none more than 2 cm in greatest dimension, with vascular invasion, or multiple tumors limited to one lobe, any more than 2 cm in greatest dimension, with or without vascular invasion |
|  |  |  | T4 Multiple tumors in more than one lobe or tumors involves a major branch of portal or hepatic veins or invasion of adjacent organs other than the gallbladder, or perforation of visceral peritoneum |
| 6 | 2002 | 2003 | T1 Solitary tumor without vascular invasion |
|  |  |  | T2 Solitary tumor with vascular invasion, or multiple tumors, none >5 cm |
|  |  |  | T3 Multiple tumors, any >5 cm (T3a), or tumors involving major branch of portal or hepatic veins |
|  |  |  | T4 Tumors with direct invasion of adjacent organs other than the gallbladder, or with perforation of visceral peritoneum |
| 7 | 2009 | 2010 | T1 Single tumor without vascular invasionc |
|  |  |  | T2 Single tumor with vascular invasion, or multiple tumors, none >5 cm |
|  |  |  | T3 Multiple tumors, any >5 cm (T3a), or tumors involving major branch of portal or hepatic veins (T3b) |
|  |  |  | T4 Tumors with direct invasion of adjacent organs other than the gallbladder, or perforation of visceral peritoneum |

changes from a relatively "benign" behavior to a more aggressive progression.[8, 18, 19, 36, 55]. This 3-cm cutoff seems to be the best point to define SHCC [8]. Other scholars have also found the relationship between tumor size and DNA ploidy [37] .

The tumor size definition in the T stage of the seventh edition of the AJCC might need to be re-evaluated by a large scale, multi-center prognostic analysis on biological stage, clinical stage, and other pathological observations. The size of HCC of 3 cm might have to be re-considered as an important factor.

## 2.4 Can SHCC Be Cured by RFA Basing on Its Pathological Characteristics?

Buscarini et al. in 1992 and Rossi et al. in 1993 first reported that radiofrequency ablation (RFA) is an easy-to-operate and minimally invasive technique that provides an effective local treatment. Subsequently, Shiina et al. [102] reported in cases with a small number (<3 nodules) of small size (<3 cm in diameter) hepatocellular carcinomas (HCC), RFA was superior to the conventional HCC treatments of percutaneous ethanol injection therapy and surgical resection in terms of recurrence, complications, and survival rates. However, some tumors remain difficult to treat with RFA because these tumors cannot be visualized or are adjacent to intestinal loops or main bile ducts, which might be damaged by the treatment.

RFA can be performed percutaneously, laparoscopically, or during laparotomy and can replace surgical resection in selected patients with SHCC. However, long-term results are difficult to ascertain, because the majority of reports evaluated success in terms of tumor necrosis and few data are available on overall and disease-free survivals of patients. In this book chapter, we primarily focus on the effectiveness of RFA on SHCC based on its pathological characteristics. We also discuss protocols and new developments in ablation techniques.

### 2.4.1 Development of RFA in SHCC Therapy

RFA is a physical thermal ablation technique which induces thermal injury to tissues through electromagnetic energy deposition. The temperature can reach to 90–120 °C by agitation resulting in frictional heat around the electrode. This leads to immediate tissue death and thermal coagulation necrosis [103]. There are three stages of development of RFA in clinical treatment of SHCC. In the first stage (during the early 1990s), only a single and solid-center needle electrode was used, and a very small diameter of ablative region of about 1.6 cm was achieved. It was not widely adopted in clinical practice because of the limited ablative region and lack of experience in its application. It the second stage (the mid-1990s), a multiple electrode, the LeVeen electrode, and an internally cooled needle electrode were developed, which led to an increase in diameter of the ablative region to 3.5–5.0 cm. These developments made very significant improvement in the therapeutic effectiveness, and RFA gradually becomes widely used in the treatment of SHCC and other tumors. As a result, RFA gradually replaced other forms of ablative therapies and became the focus of attention. In the last stage, a new generation of electrode was invented, which integrated two-different mechanisms: a combined cluster needle electrode and a saline enhanced electrode. New electrodes used clinically for SHCC now include the expandable LeVeen (Boston Scientific Corp., Natick, MA, USA) and the monopolar Cool-tip (Covidien, Boulder, CO, USA). The LeVeen needle contains an array with diameters of 20, 30, 35, or 40 mm, and the Cool-tip needle includes a 10-mm and a 20-mm non-insulated tip, respectively. The selection of needle electrodes depends on tumor size. The selection of needle electrodes should also take into consideration the condition of the surrounding hepatic tissues to ensure a sufficient ablative margin. Masayoshi et al. [104] proposed a solution in the selection of an electrode, which can produce a wider area of ablation than what is normally required.

Over the past two decades, radiofrequency ablation (RFA) has evolved into an important therapeutic tool for treatment of SHCC. In 1996, Rossi et al. [105] first reported the long-term survival rates of RFA for SHCC. Thirty-nine patients with SHCC ≤ 3.0 cm in diameter were enrolled for RFA therapy. The overall 1-, 3-, and 5-year survival rates were 97 %, 68%, and 40 %, respectively. RFA has gradually been accepted in the treatment of SHCC, although for some clinicians, the preferred treatment for SHCC is still surgical resection and liver transplantation. RFA has significant advantages over surgery which include the following: (1) it is minimally invasive procedure and it has a high efficacy. It only takes about 10 min to ablate a tumor ≤ 3.0 cm completely. The wound is small, and the recovery is rapid; (2) it has only a relatively small impact on liver function and quality of life; (3) it is safe. A study which included 2320 patients with 3530 HCC tumors reported that the mortality after RFA was 0.3 % [106]; (4) it has a very low rate of complication; (5) it is cost-effective and has easy operability, the procedure can be done in a day clinic; and (6) the necrotic tumor tissues after treatment can become a source of autogenous vaccine, which enhances the immune response to cancer.

## 2.4.2 Pathological Characteristics and Other Factors Which Impact on Prognosis of RFA for SHCC

RFA offers a new option of curative treatment for SHCC. The initial results are encouraging, and it can be used in patients when surgical resection or liver transplantation is contraindicated because of poor general condition of patients. In most studies, the initial complete tumor response rates for small HCCs ≤ 3 cm following RFA have been reported to be 90–95 %. The estimated 3- and 5-year overall and disease-free survival rates were 67.0 % and 40.1 % and 68.0 and 38.0 %, respectively. The local tumor progression rates were 10–20 %. There are factors which affect good outcomes of RFA. There is no controversy that the patient's own body mass index (BMI),

which reflects technical difficulty in carrying out RFA, is significantly associated with results of RFA therapy for SHCC. Other factors include the following:

1. Tumor location and methods of RFA: when compared to surgical resection, percutaneous RFA is more likely to result in residual tumors, especially when the lesions are located at some specific sites of the liver, e.g., underneath the liver capsule, adjacent to the gallbladder, or under the diaphragm. Laparoscopic approach appears to be the safest and most effective method to treat small tumors on the liver surface and offers the additional advantages of laparoscopic ultrasound, which provides a good resolution to show the number and location of liver tumors. Although more invasive, open RFA can be performed and the direction of puncture of the RF needle can be better selected than the laparoscopic approach, especially for lesions located close to the gallbladder or in contact with the diaphragm.

2. Tumor size: in a report coming from Japan, 183 patients with a solitary HCC of 3 cm or less were treated either with hepatic resection (HR) (n = 101) or RFA (n = 82) as a first-line treatment. There were no significant differences between the two groups for HCC of 2 cm or less. In patients treated with RFA, a tumor size of more than 2 cm was the only independent prognostic factor of a worse disease-free survival (risk ratio = 1.832, $P = 0.039$) [107].

3. Serum albumin: Peng et al. reported that in 224 patients with a solitary HCC ≤ 5 cm and with a liver background of Child-Pugh class A treated with RFA between November 1999 and June 2007, the overall 5-, 7-, 10-year survival rates were 59.8 %, 55.2 %, 33.9 %, respectively. The median overall survival was 76.1 months. Complete ablation was achieved in 216 patients (96.4 %). Serum albumin was the only factor which significantly impacted recurrence-free and tumor-free survivals ($P = 0.008$, 0.002, respectively) [108].

4. Serum alpha fetoprotein (AFP) and age: in a study from South Korea, 570 patients with

674 early-stage HCCs were treated with percutaneous RFA. The primary technique effectiveness rate was 96.7 %. The cumulative survival rates at 1, 2, 3, 4, and 5 years were 95.2 %, 82.9 %, 69.5 %, 60.8 %, and 58.0 %, respectively. Patients with Child-Pugh class A cirrhosis, younger age (≤58 years), or low AFP level (≤100 microg/L) demonstrated better survival results (P<0.05). The Child-Pugh class, age, and AFP level before RFA were significant prognostic predictors of long-term survival [109].

5. Endothelial cell-specific molecule 1 (ESM-1): in a study which included 150 patients with early HCC treated with RFA, ESM-1 expression by HCC stromal endothelial cells was observed in 58 patients (40 %) and it was associated with higher serum AFP levels, larger tumors, and more frequent expression of EpCAM (a surrogate marker of activation of Wnt-ß-catenin pathway). The two independent predictive factors of overall recurrence were serum AFP (HR 1.11, p=0.045) and ESM-1 expression (HR 1.56 [1.004; 2.43], p=0.048). Thus, ESM-1 expression was an independent predictive factor of early recurrence (HR 1.81 [1.02; 3.21], p=0.042) [110].

6. High serum hyaluronic acid and HBV viral load have been reported to be the main prognostic factors of local recurrence after complete radiofrequency ablation of hepatitis-B-related small HCC [111].

7. Age: a multivariate analysis on patients with HCV-related SHCC who were treated with RFA showed age of 75 years or more [relative hazard (RH) 1.61, p=0.019] and a serum albumin level of less than 3.5 g/dL (RH 1.61, p=0.016), which were significant factors of a decrease in overall survival. Furthermore, a serum albumin level of less than 3.5 g/dL (RH 1.50, p=0.003) was the only significant factor of decrease in recurrence-free survival [112].

8. Neutrophil-to-lymphocyte ratio (NLR): an elevated preoperative NLR has been reported to be a prognostic factor for SHCC patients after RFA treatment. Multivariate analysis showed that the postoperative change in NLR, but not the preoperative NLR, was an independent prognostic factor of both overall survival (P<0.001, HR=2.39, 95%CI 1.53–3.72) and recurrence-free survival (P=0.003, HR=1.69, 95%CI 1.87–8.24). The postoperative change in NLR was an independent prognostic factor, and patients with a decrease in NLR had better survival than those with an increase in NLR [113].

## Conclusion

In conclusion, RFA is safe and effective for treating SHCC, with the advantages of having less complication, easy operation, and rapid recovery. There is no difference in disease-free survival and overall survival, and RFA and surgical resection in patients with SHCC are safe and effective. However, the pathological characteristics of SHCC with more aggressive behavior such as DNA aneuploidy, microvascular invasion, microscopic satellites, poor differentiation, capsular invasion, tumor location as well as macroscopic growth patterns, can influence the long-term treatment results for both RFA and surgical resection.

## References

1. Tang ZY. Subclinical hepatocellular carcinoma: Historical aspects and general consideration. In: Tang ZY, editor. Subclinical hepatocellular carcinoma. Berlin: Springer; 1985. p. 1–11.
2. Zhaoyou T, Yeqin Y, Zhiying L, et al. Small hepatocellular carcinoma: clinical analysis of 30 cases. Chin Med J (Engl). 1979;92(7):455–62.
3. Wu MC, Chen H, Zhang XH, et al. Primary hepatic carcinoma resection over 18 years. Chin Med J (Engl). 1980;93(10):723–8.
4. Llovet JM, Bru C, Bruix J. Prognosis of hepatocellular carcinoma: the BCLC staging classification. Semin Liver Dis. 1999;19(3):329–38.
5. Okuda K, Nakashima T, Obata H, et al. Clinicopathological studies of minute hepatocellular carcinoma. Analysis of 20 cases, including 4 with hepatic resection. Gastroenterology. 1977;73(1):109–15.
6. Kanematsu T, Sonoda T, Takenaka K, et al. The value of ultrasound in the diagnosis and treatment of small hepatocellular carcinoma. Br J Surg. 1985;72(1):23–5.
7. Kondo Y, Niwa Y, Akikusa B, et al. A histopathologic study of early hepatocellular carcinoma. Cancer. 1983;52(4):687–92.

8. Cong WM, Wu MC. The biopathologic characteristics of DNA content of hepatocellular carcinomas. Cancer. 1990;66(3):498–501.

9. Libbrecht L, Severi T, Cassiman D, et al. Glypican-3 expression distinguishes small hepatocellular carcinomas from cirrhosis, dysplastic nodules, and focal nodular hyperplasia-like nodules. Am J Surg Pathol. 2006;30(11):1405–11.

10. Aishima S, Nishihara Y, Kuroda Y, et al. Histologic characteristics and prognostic significance in small hepatocellular carcinoma with biliary differentiation: subdivision and comparison with ordinary hepatocellular carcinoma. Am J Surg Pathol. 2007;31(5):783–91.

11. Okuwaki Y, Nakazawa T, Shibuya A, et al. Intrahepatic distant recurrence after radiofrequency ablation for a single small hepatocellular carcinoma: risk factors and patterns. J Gastroenterol. 2008;43(1):71–8.

12. Kudo M. Atypical large well-differentiated hepatocellular carcinoma with benign nature: a new clinical entity. Intervirology. 2004;47(3-5):227–37.

13. Arii S, Yamaoka Y, Futagawa S, et al. Results of surgical and nonsurgical treatment for small-sized hepatocellular carcinomas: a retrospective and nationwide survey in Japan. The Liver Cancer Study Group of Japan. Hepatology. 2000;32(6):1224–9.

14. Vauthey JN, Lauwers GY, Esnaola NF, et al. Simplified staging for hepatocellular carcinoma. J Clin Oncol. 2002;20(6):1527–36.

15. Forner A, Vilana R, Ayuso C, et al. Diagnosis of hepatic nodules 20 mm or smaller in cirrhosis: prospective validation of the noninvasive diagnostic criteria for hepatocellular carcinoma. Hepatology. 2008;47(1):97–104.

16. Farinati F, Sergio A, Baldan A, et al. Early and very early hepatocellular carcinoma: when and how much do staging and choice of treatment really matter? A multi-center study. BMC Cancer. 2009;9:33.

17. Cong W, Wu M, Wang Y, et al. Primary liver tumors in China. Oncol Rep. 1997;4(3):649–52.

18. Lu XY, Xi T, Lau WY, et al. Pathobiological features of small hepatocellular carcinoma: correlation between tumor size and biological behavior. J Cancer Res Clin Oncol. 2011;137(4):567–75.

19. Cong WM. Clinicopathologic features of small hepatocellular carcinoma – an analysis of ninety-three cases. Zhonghua Zhong Liu Za Zhi. 1993;15(5):372–4.

20. Pawlik TM, Delman KA, Vauthey JN, et al. Tumor size predicts vascular invasion and histologic grade: Implications for selection of surgical treatment for hepatocellular carcinoma. Liver Transpl. 2005;11(9):1086–92.

21. LCSGO. Classification of primary liver cancer. Tokyo: Kanehara Press Co; 1997.

22. Matsui O, Kadoya M, Kameyama T, et al. Benign and malignant nodules in cirrhotic livers: distinction based on blood supply. Radiology. 1991;178(2):493–7.

23. Mazzaferro V, Regalia E, Doci R, et al. Liver transplantation for the treatment of small hepatocellular carcinomas in patients with cirrhosis. N Engl J Med. 1996;334(11):693–9.

24. Nathan H, Hyder O, Mayo SC, et al. Surgical therapy for early hepatocellular carcinoma in the modern era: a 10-year SEER-medicare analysis. Ann Surg. 2013;258(6):1022–7.

25. Llovet JM, Bruix J, Fuster J, et al. Liver transplantation for small hepatocellular carcinoma: the tumor-node-metastasis classification does not have prognostic power. Hepatology. 1998;27(6):1572–7.

26. Llovet JM, Fuster J, Bruix J. Intention-to-treat analysis of surgical treatment for early hepatocellular carcinoma: resection versus transplantation. Hepatology. 1999;30(6):1434–40.

27. Llovet JM, Chen Y, Wurmbach E, et al. A molecular signature to discriminate dysplastic nodules from early hepatocellular carcinoma in HCV cirrhosis. Gastroenterology. 2006;131(6):1758–67.

28. Llovet JM, Burroughs A, Bruix J. Hepatocellular carcinoma. Lancet. 2003;362(9399):1907–17.

29. Sakamoto M, Hirohashi S. Natural history and prognosis of adenomatous hyperplasia and early hepatocellular carcinoma: multi-institutional analysis of 53 nodules followed up for more than 6 months and 141 patients with single early hepatocellular carcinoma treated by surgical resection or percutaneous ethanol injection. Jpn J Clin Oncol. 1998;28(10):604–8.

30. Takayama T, Makuuchi M, Hirohashi S, et al. Early hepatocellular carcinoma as an entity with a high rate of surgical cure. Hepatology. 1998;28(5):1241–6.

31. Bruix J, Sherman M. Practice Guidelines Committee AaFTSOLD. Management of hepatocellular carcinoma. Hepatology. 2005;42(5):1208–36.

32. Bruix J, Sherman M. American Association for the Study of Liver Diseases. Management of hepatocellular carcinoma: an update. Hepatology. 2011;53(3):1020–2.

33. Sakamoto M. Pathology of early hepatocellular carcinoma. Hepatol Res. 2007;37 Suppl 2:S135–8.

34. Sakamoto M. Early HCC: diagnosis and molecular markers. J Gastroenterol. 2009;44 Suppl 19: 108–11.

35. Kim SJ, Lee KK, Kim DG. Tumor size predicts the biological behavior and influence of operative modalities in hepatocellular carcinoma. Hepatogastroenterology. 2010;57(97):121–6.

36. Cong Wm WM. Significance of clinicopathology in quantitative measurement of DNA content in hepatocellular carcinoma. J Med Coll PLA. 1988;3: 153–6.

37. Ng IO, Lai EC, Ho JC, et al. Flow cytometric analysis of DNA ploidy in hepatocellular carcinoma. Am J Clin Pathol. 1994;102(1):80–6.

38. Kojiro M, Wanless IR, Alves V, et al. International Consensus Group for Hepatocellular Neoplasiathe International Consensus Group for Hepatocellular N. Pathologic diagnosis of early hepatocellular carcinoma: a report of the international consensus

group for hepatocellular neoplasia. Hepatology. 2009;49(2):658–64.

39. Llovet JM, Fuster J, Bruix J, et al. The Barcelona approach: diagnosis, staging, and treatment of hepatocellular carcinoma. Liver Transpl. 2004;10(2 Suppl 1):S115–20.

40. Tsuda H, Hirohashi S, Shimosato Y, et al. Clonal origin of atypical adenomatous hyperplasia of the liver and clonal identity with hepatocellular carcinoma. Gastroenterology. 1988;95(6):1664–6.

41. Takayama T, Makuuchi M, Hirohashi S, et al. Malignant transformation of adenomatous hyperplasia to hepatocellular carcinoma. Lancet. 1990;336(8724):1150–3.

42. Sakamoto M, Hirohashi S, Shimosato Y. Early stages of multistep hepatocarcinogenesis: adenomatous hyperplasia and early hepatocellular carcinoma. Hum Pathol. 1991;22(2):172–8.

43. Liver Cancer Study Group of Japan. Primary liver cancer in Japan. Clinicopathologic features and results of surgical treatment. Ann Surg. 1990;211(3):277–87.

44. Livraghi T, Bolondi L, Buscarini L, et al. No treatment, resection and ethanol injection in hepatocellular carcinoma: a retrospective analysis of survival in 391 patients with cirrhosis. Italian Cooperative HCC Study Group. J Hepatol. 1995;22(5):522–6.

45. Ryder SD, British Society of Group. Guidelines for the diagnosis and treatment of hepatocellular carcinoma (HCC) in adults. Gut. 2003;52(3):1–8.

46. Forner A, Hessheimer AJ, Isabel Real M, et al. Treatment of hepatocellular carcinoma. Crit Rev Oncol Hematol. 2006;60(2):89–98.

47. Edge SB, Byrd DR, Carducci MA. American Joint Committee on Cancer (AJCC) Cancer staging manual. New York: Springer; 2009.

48. Kunavisarut T, Kak I, Macmillan C, et al. Immunohistochemical analysis based Ep-ICD subcellular localization index (ESLI) is a novel marker for metastatic papillary thyroid microcarcinoma. BMC Cancer. 2012;12:523.

49. Edge SB, Byrd DR, Compton CC. AJCC Cancer staging manual. New York: Springer; 2010. p. 347–76.

50. Laudano MA, Klafter FE, Katz M, et al. Pathological tumour diameter predicts risk of conventional subtype in small renal cortical tumours. BJU Int. 2008;102(10):1385–8.

51. Saito H, Osaki T, Murakami D, et al. Macroscopic tumor size as a simple prognostic indicator in patients with gastric cancer. Am J Surg. 2006;192(3):296–300.

52. Zy T. Primary liver cancer. Shanghai: Shanghai Scientific & Technical Publishers; 1981.

53. Ebara M, Ohto M, Shinagawa T, et al. Natural history of minute hepatocellular carcinoma smaller than three centimeters complicating cirrhosis. A study in 22 patients. Gastroenterology. 1986;90(2):289–98.

54. Kanai T, Hirohashi S, Upton MP, et al. Pathology of small hepatocellular carcinoma. A proposal for a new gross classification. Cancer. 1987;60(4):810–9.

55. Cong WM. Clinical studies on pathobiological characteristics of early hepatocellular carcinoma. Zhonghua Wai Ke Za Zhi. 1991;29(6):341–4, 396.

56. Moribe T, Iizuka N, Miura T, et al. Methylation of multiple genes as molecular markers for diagnosis of a small, well-differentiated hepatocellular carcinoma. Int J Cancer. 2009;125(2):388–97.

57. Kojiro M. 'Nodule-in-nodule' appearance in hepatocellular carcinoma: its significance as a morphologic marker of dedifferentiation. Intervirology. 2004;47(3–5):179–83.

58. Lam VW, Ng KK, Chok KS, et al. Incomplete ablation after radiofrequency ablation of hepatocellular carcinoma: analysis of risk factors and prognostic factors. Ann Surg Oncol. 2008;15(3):782–90.

59. Ueno S, Kubo F, Sakoda M, et al. Efficacy of anatomic resection vs nonanatomic resection for small nodular hepatocellular carcinoma based on gross classification. J Hepatobiliary Pancreat Surg. 2008;15(5):493–500.

60. Vilana R, Bruix J, Bru C, et al. Tumor size determines the efficacy of percutaneous ethanol injection for the treatment of small hepatocellular carcinoma. Hepatology. 1992;16(2):353–7.

61. Kojiro M, Nakashima O. Histopathologic evaluation of hepatocellular carcinoma with special reference to small early stage tumors. Semin Liver Dis. 1999;19(3):287–96.

62. Shimada M, Rikimaru T, Hamatsu T, et al. The role of macroscopic classification in nodular-type hepatocellular carcinoma. Am J Surg. 2001;182(2): 177–82.

63. Hu RH, Lee PH, Chang YC, et al. Prognostic factors for hepatocellular carcinoma < or = 3 cm in diameter. Hepatogastroenterology. 2003;50(54):2043–8.

64. Shimozawa N, Hanazaki K. Longterm prognosis after hepatic resection for small hepatocellular carcinoma. J Am Coll Surg. 2004;198(3):356–65.

65. Wu FS, Zhao WH, Liang TB, et al. Survival factors after resection of small hepatocellular carcinoma. Hepatobiliary Pancreat Dis Int. 2005;4(3):379–84.

66. Marelli L, Grasso A, Pleguezuelo M, et al. Tumour size and differentiation in predicting recurrence of hepatocellular carcinoma after liver transplantation: external validation of a new prognostic score. Ann Surg Oncol. 2008;15(12):3503–11.

67. Cancer CSOL. Clinical diagnosis and staging of primary liver cancer. Chin J Hepatol. 2001;9:324.

68. Kudo M, Izumi N, Kokudo N, et al. Management of hepatocellular carcinoma in Japan: Consensus-Based Clinical Practice Guidelines proposed by the Japan Society of Hepatology (JSH) 2010 updated version. Dig Dis. 2011;29(3):339–64.

69. Tiong L, Maddern GJ. Systematic review and meta-analysis of survival and disease recurrence after radiofrequency ablation for hepatocellular carcinoma. Br J Surg. 2011;98(9):1210–24.

70. Cabrera R, Nelson DR. Review article: the management of hepatocellular carcinoma. Aliment Pharmacol Ther. 2010;31(4):461–76.

71. Memon K, Kulik L, Lewandowski RJ, et al. Radiographic response to locoregional therapy in hepatocellular carcinoma predicts patient survival times. Gastroenterology. 2011;141(2):526–35, 535 e521-522.

72. Hermanek P, Sobin LH. TNM classification of malignant tumours. Berlin: Springer; 1987.

73. Sobin LH, Wittekind C. TNM classification of malignant tumours. New York: Wiley-Liss; 1997.

74. Izumi R, Shimizu K, Ii T, et al. Prognostic factors of hepatocellular carcinoma in patients undergoing hepatic resection. Gastroenterology. 1994;106(3): 720–7.

75. Staudacher C, Chiappa A, Biella F, et al. Validation of the modified TNM-Izumi classification for hepatocellular carcinoma. Tumori. 2000;86(1):8–11.

76. Chiappa A, Zbar AP, Podda M, et al. Prognostic value of the modified TNM (Izumi) classification of hepatocellular carcinoma in 53 cirrhotic patients undergoing resection. Hepatogastroenterology. 2001;48(37):229–34.

77. Kudo M, Chung H, Osaki Y. Prognostic staging system for hepatocellular carcinoma (CLIP score): its value and limitations, and a proposal for a new staging system, the Japan Integrated Staging Score (JIS score). J Gastroenterol. 2003;38(3):207–15.

78. Kondo F, Hirooka N, Wada K, et al. Morphological clues for the diagnosis of small hepatocellular carcinomas. Virchows Arch A Pathol Anat Histopathol. 1987;411(1):15–21.

79. Nagao T, Nagashima I, Inoue S, et al. Hepatic resection for minute hepatocellular carcinoma. Surg Today. 1992;22(2):110–4.

80. Nakashima O, Sugihara S, Kage M, et al. Pathomorphologic characteristics of small hepatocellular carcinoma: a special reference to small hepatocellular carcinoma with indistinct margins. Hepatology. 1995;22(1):101–5.

81. Ikai I, Arii S, Kojiro M, et al. Reevaluation of prognostic factors for survival after liver resection in patients with hepatocellular carcinoma in a Japanese nationwide survey. Cancer. 2004;101(4):796–802.

82. Ando E, Kuromatsu R, Tanaka M, et al. Surveillance program for early detection of hepatocellular carcinoma in Japan: results of specialized department of liver disease. J Clin Gastroenterol. 2006;40(10):942–8.

83. Minagawa M, Ikai I, Matsuyama Y, et al. Staging of hepatocellular carcinoma: assessment of the Japanese TNM and AJCC/UICC TNM systems in a cohort of 13,772 patients in Japan. Ann Surg. 2007;245(6):909–22.

84. Livraghi T, Meloni F, Di Stasi M, et al. Sustained complete response and complications rates after radiofrequency ablation of very early hepatocellular carcinoma in cirrhosis: Is resection still the treatment of choice? Hepatology. 2008;47(1):82–9.

85. Takayama T, Makuuchi M, Hasegawa K. Single HCC smaller than 2 cm: surgery or ablation?: surgeon's perspective. J Hepatobiliary Pancreat Sci. 2010;17(4):422–4.

86. Di Tommaso L, Destro A, Fabbris V, et al. Diagnostic accuracy of clathrin heavy chain staining in a marker panel for the diagnosis of small hepatocellular carcinoma. Hepatology. 2011;53(5):1549–57.

87. Yamashita Y, Tsuijita E, Takeishi K, et al. Predictors for microinvasion of small hepatocellular carcinoma </= 2 cm. Ann Surg Oncol. 2012;19(6):2027–34.

88. Kojiro M. Focus on dysplastic nodules and early hepatocellular carcinoma: an Eastern point of view. Liver Transpl. 2004;10(2 Suppl 1):S3–8.

89. Nakashima Y, Nakashima O, Tanaka M, et al. Portal vein invasion and intrahepatic micrometastasis in small hepatocellular carcinoma by gross type. Hepatol Res. 2003;26(2):142–7.

90. Sasaki Y, Imaoka S, Ishiguro S, et al. Clinical features of small hepatocellular carcinomas as assessed by histologic grades. Surgery. 1996;119(3):252–60.

91. Desmet VJ. East-West pathology agreement on precancerous liver lesions and early hepatocellular carcinoma. Hepatology. 2009;49(2):355–7.

92. Kondo F. Histological features of early hepatocellular carcinomas and their developmental process: for daily practical clinical application : Hepatocellular carcinoma. Hepatol Int. 2009;3(1):283–93.

93. Park YN. Update on precursor and early lesions of hepatocellular carcinomas. Arch Pathol Lab Med. 2011;135(6):704–15.

94. Di Tommaso L, Sangiovanni A, Borzio M, et al. Advanced precancerous lesions in the liver. Best Pract Res Clin Gastroenterol. 2013;27(2):269–84.

95. Kojiro M. Diagnostic discrepancy of early hepatocellular carcinoma between Japan and West. Hepatol Res. 2007;37 Suppl 2:S121–4.

96. Bolondi L, Gaiani S, Celli N, et al. Characterization of small nodules in cirrhosis by assessment of vascularity: the problem of hypovascular hepatocellular carcinoma. Hepatology. 2005;42(1):27–34.

97. Henderson JM, Sherman M, Tavill A, et al. AHPBA/AJCC consensus conference on staging of hepatocellular carcinoma: consensus statement. HPB (Oxford). 2003;5(4):243–50.

98. Lu W, Dong J, Huang Z, et al. Comparison of four current staging systems for Chinese patients with hepatocellular carcinoma undergoing curative resection: Okuda, CLIP TNM and CUPI. J Gastroenterol Hepatol. 2008;23(12):1874–8.

99. Greene F, Fleming I, Fritz A, et al. AJCC cancer staging manual. Chicago: Springer, 2010. p 435.

100. Forner A, Reig ME, De Lope CR, et al. Current strategy for staging and treatment: the BCLC update and future prospects. Semin Liver Dis. 2010;30(1): 61–74.

101. Cong WM, Wu MC. Small hepatocellular carcinoma-current and future approaches. Hepatol Int. 2013;7(3):805–12.

102. Shiina S, Teratani T, Obi S, et al. Nonsurgical treatment of hepatocellular carcinoma: from percutaneous ethanol injection therapy and percutaneous microwave coagulation therapy to radiofrequency ablation. Oncology. 2002;62 Suppl 1:64–8.

103. Lencioni R, Crocetti L, Cioni D, et al. Percutaneous radiofrequency ablation of hepatic colorectal metastases: technique, indications, results, and new promises. Invest Radiol. 2004;39(11):689–97.

104. Masayoshi T, Wakui N, Sumino Y. Use of radiofrequency ablation in the treatment of hepatocellular carcinoma: Experience of ablation protocols. Exp Ther Med. 2012;4(6):959–61.

105. Rossi S, Di Stasi M, Buscarini E, et al. Percutaneous RF interstitial thermal ablation in the treatment of hepatic cancer. AJR Am J Roentgenol. 1996;167(3):759–68.

106. Livraghi T, Solbiati L, Meloni MF, et al. Treatment of focal liver tumors with percutaneous radiofrequency ablation: complications encountered in a multicenter study. Radiology. 2003;226(2):441–51.

107. Imai K, Beppu T, Chikamoto A, et al. Comparison between hepatic resection and radiofrequency ablation as first-line treatment for solitary small-sized hepatocellular carcinoma of 3 cm or less. Hepatol Res. 2013;43(8):853–64.

108. Peng ZW, Zhang YJ, Chen MS, et al. Radiofrequency ablation as first-line treatment for small solitary hepatocellular carcinoma: long-term results. Eur J Surg Oncol. 2010;36(11):1054–60.

109. Choi D, Lim HK, Rhim H, et al. Percutaneous radiofrequency ablation for early-stage hepatocellular carcinoma as a first-line treatment: long-term results and prognostic factors in a large single-institution series. Eur Radiol. 2007;17(3):684–92.

110. Ziol M, Sutton A, Calderaro J, et al. ESM-1 expression in stromal cells is predictive of recurrence after radiofrequency ablation in early hepatocellular carcinoma. J Hepatol. 2013;59(6):1264–70.

111. Xia F, Lai EC, Lau WY, et al. High serum hyaluronic acid and HBV viral load are main prognostic factors of local recurrence after complete radiofrequency ablation of hepatitis B-related small hepatocellular carcinoma. Ann Surg Oncol. 2012;19(4):1284–91.

112. Toshikuni N, Takuma Y, Goto T, et al. Prognostic factors in hepatitis C patients with a single small hepatocellular carcinoma after radiofrequency ablation. Hepatogastroenterology. 2012;59(120):2361–6.

113. Dan J, Zhang Y, Peng Z, et al. Postoperative neutrophil-to-lymphocyte ratio change predicts survival of patients with small hepatocellular carcinoma undergoing radiofrequency ablation. PLoS One. 2013;8(3), e58184.

# Radiofrequency Ablation Systems and Operating Mechanisms

**3**

Yaojun Zhang

## 3.1 Introduction

In the past two decades, local ablative technique has become an important therapeutic approach for small hepatocellular carcinoma (HCC). In those various therapies, radiofrequency ablation (RFA) has attracted the greatest interest from surgeons due to its satisfactory effectiveness and safety in management of HCC (lesion ≤5.0 cm in diameter). RFA now is regarded as a curative therapy for HCC, liver resection as well as liver transplantation [1–3].

Procedure of RFA operation involves percutaneous introduction of an electrode into the tumor location and provocation of radiofrequency energy, whereupon the temperature of the tissue increases because of microwave ionic oscillation. Tissue coagulation happens when temperature around the electrode reaches up to 60 °C approximately. Moisture evaporation occurs, and the tissue turns into complete necrosis at the temperature elevating to about 90 °C. This percutaneous procedure has demonstrated the evidence-proven effectiveness and safety and also possesses the advantages of being a minimally invasive surgery [3–6].

Y. Zhang, MD, PhD
Department of Hepatobiliary Surgery, Sun Yat-sen University Cancer Center, Guangzhou, China
e-mail: zhyaojun@mail.sysu.edu.cn

## 3.1.1 The Mechanisms of RFA

RFA was evolved from electrocautery in the 1990s and had developed into the most widely used ablation modality worldwide. During the course of RF ablation, the electrical current is applied directly at the target zone. However, at least two electrodes are required to complete an electrical circuit through the physical body. The typical modality is to insert one electrode into the body (interstitial electrode) and fix other electrode to the skin surface (dispersive electrode or grounding pads, Fig. 3.1). At that time, the patient is a part of a closed-loop circuit composed of a RF generator, an electrode needle, a large dispersive electrode, or grounding pads. An alternating electric field is created within the tissue of the patient. Because of relative higher electrical resistance of tissue in comparison with the metal electrodes, there is remarkable ionic oscillation in the target tissue adjacent to the electrode owing to the tissue ions attempting to follow the direction changes of alternating current. The ionic oscillation produces frictional heat around the electrode. The discrepancy between the small surface area of the needle electrode and the large size of the grounding pads may result to heat generation focused on and concentrated around the needle electrode, so the local temperature can achieve up to 90 °C or so [7, 8].

Elevated temperature is able to impair the cells via several ways. The primary manner of

© Springer Science+Business Media Dordrecht 2016
M. Chen et al. (eds.), *Radiofrequency Ablation for Small Hepatocellular Carcinoma*,
DOI 10.1007/978-94-017-7258-7_3

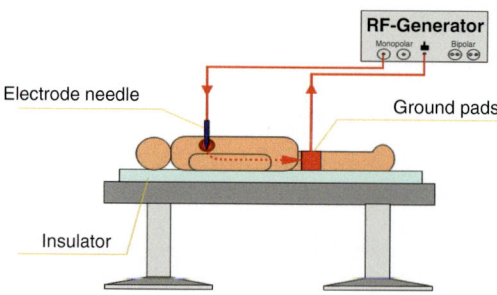

**Fig. 3.1** Schematic set up of liver RF treatment with assumed current pathways

cell death during thermal ablation for tumor is acute coagulative necrosis. When temperature is up to 41°C, it causes the blood vessel dilation and the increase of blood perfusion. Meantime, it can stimulate the production of heat-shock protein for protecting the cell from heat injury and repairing the damage tissue. Nevertheless, this temperature-stimulated protective mechanism is associated with heat intensity and heat exposure time. When temperature is up to 46°C and heat exposure is up to 10 min, irreversible necrosis of significant cell mass will produce. Cells recovery from heat injury may exhibit an increased tolerance to elevated temperatures. Temperatures at 46–52°C will attenuate the time to induce cell death and begin to trigger microvascular thrombosis, ischemia, and hypoxia. This reactive cascade cuts off the supply of cells' nutrient and leads to delayed cell necrosis. Temperatures in excess of 60°C will rapidly cause protein denaturation and melt the plasma membrane, which is essential for cells survival [7, 8].

## 3.1.2    The Development of RFA

Three periods were defined since RFA was applied to manage of HCC in clinical practice according to the development of radiofrequency electrodes. The first phase was in the early 1990s when a single and solid-center needle electrode was used in RFA and only for the lesions with a size of 1.6 cm in diameter. Therefore, it was utilized infrequently in the clinic by the restriction of ablative size. The second phase was in the middle of 1990s when the electrode was greatly

modified. Then, multiple electrodes and cooled needle electrode were invented, as represented by LeVeen electrodes (Radiotherapeutics) and internally cooled electrodes (Radionics), respectively. Both of them are capable of enlarging the ablative size to 3.5–5.0 cm in diameter with dramatic improvements of therapeutic efficacy. With the comprehensive application of RFA in the treatment of HCC, it is gradually becoming the typical measure of local ablative therapy and attracts more and more attention in the field of liver surgery. The third-generation electrodes were developed by integrating the advantages of needle electrode and saline-enhanced electrode. For example, Celon Power (Olympus) has integrated two to three kinds of the second-generation electrodes so as to further increase the ablative region to 5.0–7.0 cm in diameter. Furthermore, we can apply multi-electrode ablation system to accurately position the electrodes based on the tumor's shape, then precisely realize the "conforming ablation," all of which will additionally improve the therapeutic efficacy of RFA [9, 10].

## 3.1.3    Commonly Used Commercial Available RFA Systems

There are a variety of RFA systems commercially available today, which can be divided into three categories based on their principles: temperature-controlled, impedance-controlled, and temperature-impedance-controlled operating mechanisms. There are also many kinds of electrode needles including extendable needle, single needle, multiple-needle, and needles with intrinsic/extrinsic cycle perfusion. Each RFA system usually has several matched electrode needle types with their own advantages and disadvantages. We currently introduce the most popular commercial available RFA systems as follows: Radionics™ (Radionics Medical, Boston, MA), RITA® (Rita Medical, Mountain View, CA), Radiotherapeutics™ (Radio-Therapeutics, Sunnyvale, CA), Berchtold® (Berchtold, Tuttlingen, Germany), and Celon*POWER* system (Celon AG Medical Instruments, OLYMPUS, Japan). All of them were frequently reported in publications [11–14].

### 3.1.4 Radionics™ RF System

The Cool-tip™ System (Radionics Burlington, MA, Fig. 3.2a) works at impedance control mode and 200-W power source pulses energy delivery with frequency of 480 kHz to generate the larger ablation volumes. The exclusive feedback algorithm continuously monitors the tissue impedance and automatically adjusts the maximum energy delivery. Thermocouple at electrode tip scrutinizes the tissue temperature. Once the therapeutic cycle completed, the electrode can be repositioned to measure the temperature at ablation zone.

Their needles (Fig. 3.2b) are all straight, internally cooled electrode design. Each needle is sized 1.6 mm in diameter with a 2.0–4.0 cm active distal part (Fig. 3.2b). This RF system requires four neutral pads, two on the pelvis and one on the hind thighs, respectively. The ablative zone sized 2.5–4.0 cm in diameter can be created with single needle by one operation (Fig. 3.2b). Also, we can use three electrodes simultaneously to generate the larger ablative area sized up to 6 cm in diameter (Fig. 3.2c).

### 3.2 RITA® RF System

The Model 1500™ (RITA® Medical Systems, Mountain View, CA) is a RF system with a 150-W generator and operates at 460-kHz frequency (Fig. 3.3a). The expandable electrode (StarBurst™ XL; Rita Medical Systems) consists of an insulated outer needle sized at 2.2 mm in diameter that houses nine deployable curved tines. When the electrodes are fully extended, the maximum diameter can reach to 5 cm, which mimics the configuration of a Christmas tree (Fig. 3.3b). In order to control the generator, five of the nine prongs containing thermal sensors are responsible to measure the tip temperature. The power is controlled in accordance with an average temperature of these probes. Electrodes were progressively extended deeper into the liver parenchyma, with temperature monitoring, to represent the standard algorithm widely used with this system. The standard method allows the

maximum energy to be applied until the mean temperature reaches the threshold. Tines were deployed firstly to 2 cm at a pre-selected target temperature of 80°C, then advanced to 3 cm at a targeted temperature of 105°C, and finally extended to 4–5 cm at a targeted temperature of 110°C. The targeted temperature should be maintained for 7 min prior to measuring the post-ablation temperatures with five thermocouples. For this system, two grounding pads were required to place on the thighs.

There are also several other type needles available for RITA® RF system (Fig. 3.3a), but their ablation zone is smaller than that induced by StarBurst™ XL.

### 3.2.1 Radiotherapeutics™ RF System

The RF3000™ system (Radiotherapeutics, Sunnyvale, CA) utilizes a maximum power of 200-W generator with an operating frequency of 480 kHz (Fig. 3.4a). This system is used with a 12-prong LeVeen™ multitined array electrode (Fig. 3.4b). The 2.5-mm-diameter cannula of the electrode contains 12 retracted curved distal tines, which when fully expanded form an umbrella shape, 4.0–5.0 cm in maximum diameter, perpendicular to the axis of the probe. After the deployment of tines, the power output is initially triggered at 80 W and then escalated by 10 W every 30 s until it reaches 130 W. Without the rise of impedance over 200 Ω after 5 min at 130 W, power output is increased by 10 W every 30 s up to 190 W and is continuously maintained until either a 15-min application time elapsed or an uncontrolled impedance rise is observed. After 30 s, a second circle is started and RF energy is applied until the appearance of next uncontrolled impedance rise. In case uncontrolled impedance rise occurs at the 130-W initial power in the first 5 min, power is re-applied thereby after 30 s with 50 % reduction. Subsequent power output is escalated by 10 W every 30 s up to 190 W and is continuously maintained until either the entire 15-min application time elapsed or of next impedance rise happened. There is no need for changing the

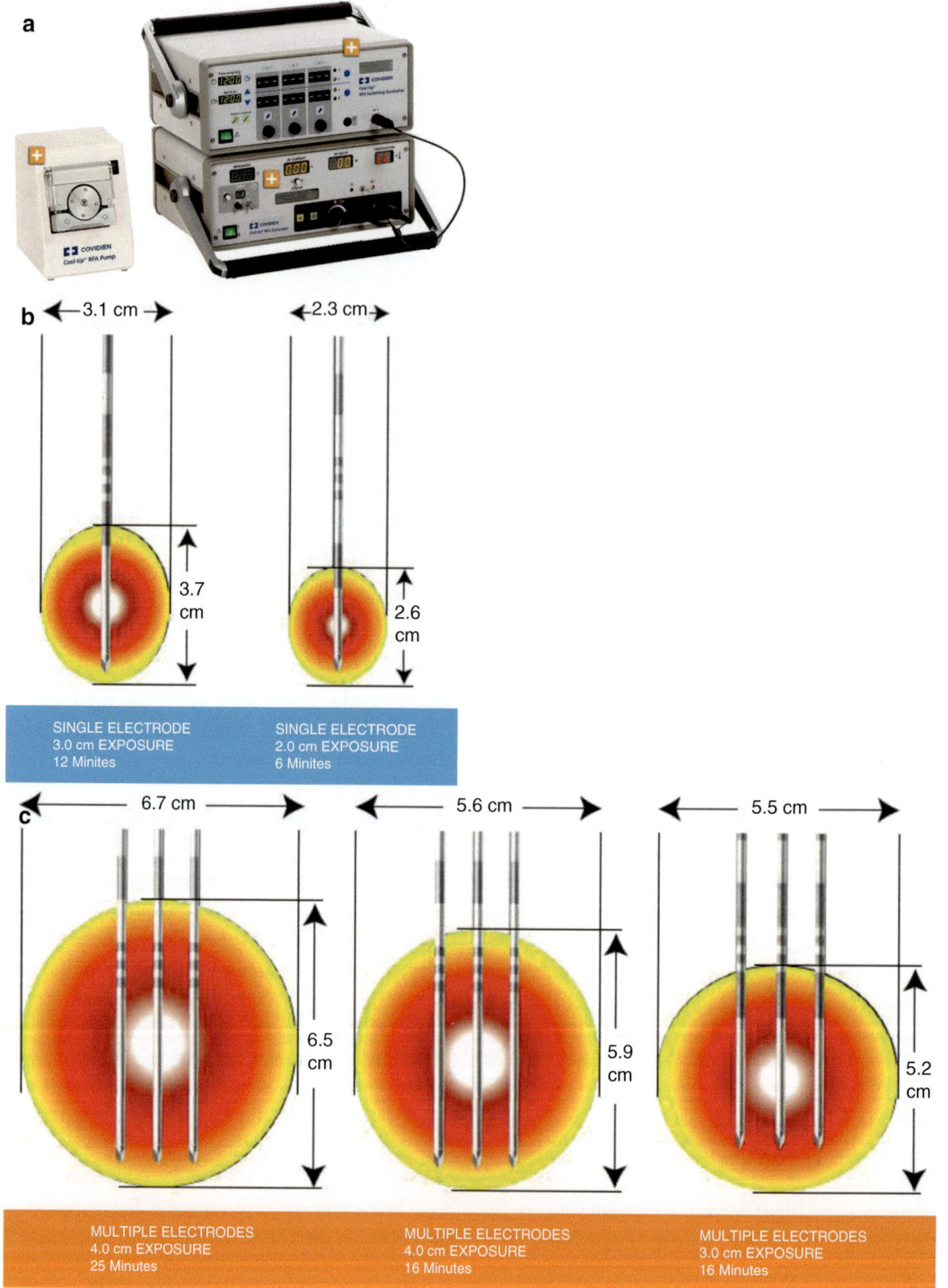

**Fig. 3.2** (**a**) The Cool-tip™ System. (**b**) The Cool-tip™ needles. (**c**) Generating a larger ablative lesion with three electrodes simultaneously

**Fig. 3.3** (**a**) The Model
1500™ (RITA® Medical
Systems, Mountain View,
CA). (**b**) The StarBurst™ XL
needle (RITA® Medical
Systems, Mountain View,
CA). (**c**) Other type of needles
for RITA® RF Systems

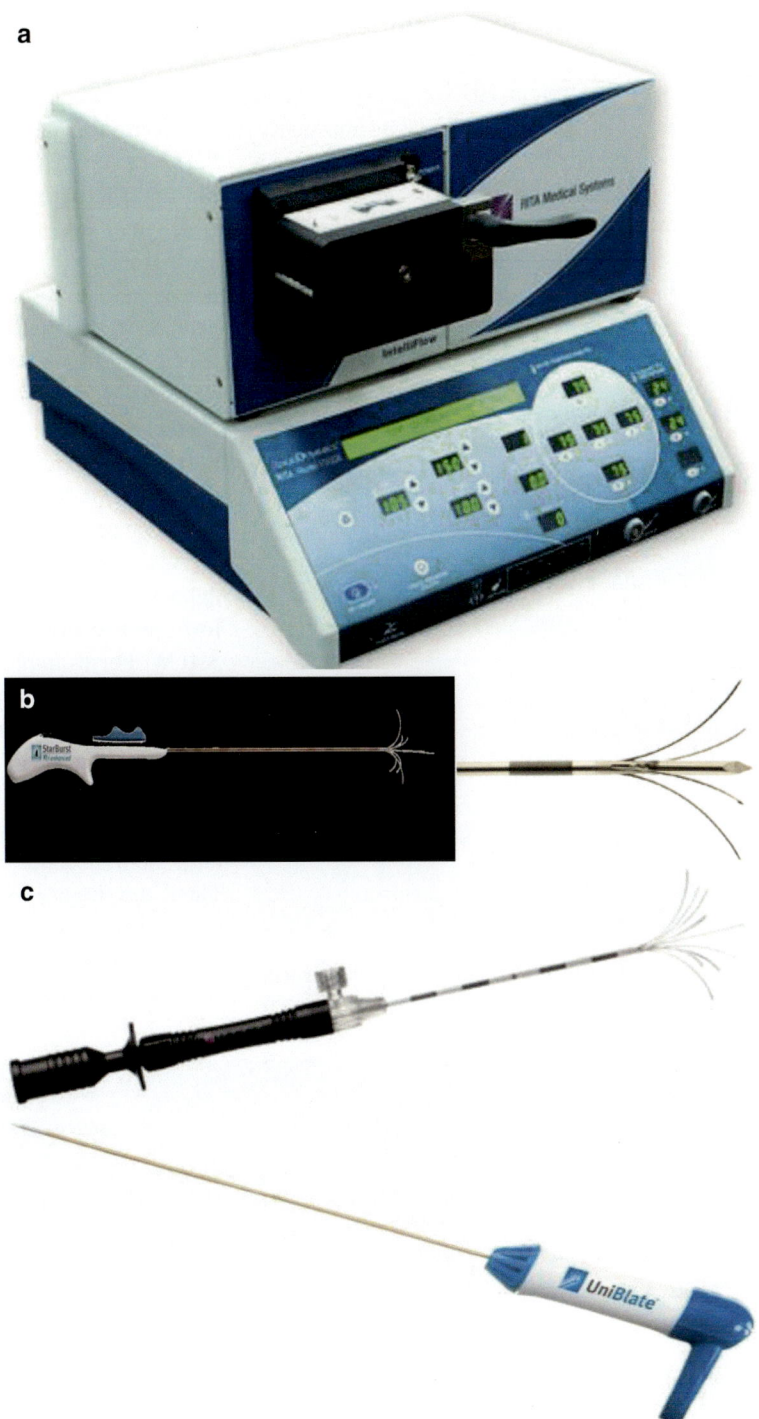

probe position; these two applications are of the capacity to create an ablation area with this system. Four grounding pads are required for each procedure, as recommended by the manufacturer. Two pads are attached on the pelvis, and one is placed on the hind thighs, respectively.

## 3.2.2 Berchtold® RF System

The system Elektrotom HiTT® 106 (Berchtold, Tuttlingen, Germany) contains an impedance-controlled monopolar 375-kHz radiofrequency generator and is capable of producing a maximum 60-W power through a 2.0-mm-diameter monopolar electrode with a 1.5-cm length active needle tip (Figs. 3.5a, b). The electrode for this saline-enhanced technique has double layer wall at its distal part with small holes on the inner wall. Infused isotonic saline flows through the hollow shaft of the electrode and permeates through the holes into the space between inner and outer walls of the needle tip. The outer wall is constructed with large rectangular apertures that permits infused fluid moves into the tissue surrounding the needle tip before and after the ablation. The flow rate of saline solution (0.9 % NaCl) is determined automatically on the basis of pre-setting power and flow range between 38 and 120 mL/h. A syringe pump (Pilot C; Fresenius Vial, Brezins, France) connected to the radiofrequency generator provides the continuous saline solution flow through six micropores on the active part of the electrode.

As a result of automatic regulation of radiofrequency power, a power curve is generated in the low impedance range between 100 and 350 W. For example, for more than 350 W, the radiofrequency power is automatically decreased in accordance with a constant voltage curve to ensure the lower impedance range. If the impedance exceeds the programmed value of $700 \pm 50$ W, radiofrequency power will be reduced to 5W until the impedance decreases to $400 \pm 50$ below. Then the higher power—the nominal power selected prior to beginning—is switched on again to continue the power curve in the lower impedance range of $300 \pm 100$ W. This control mecha-

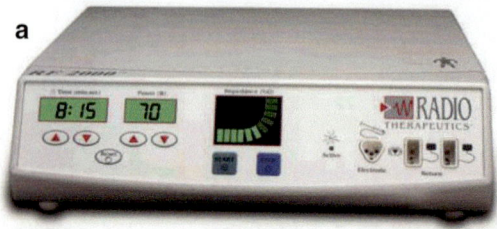

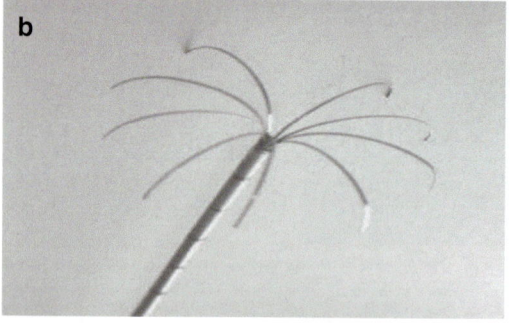

**Fig. 3.4** (**a**) The RF3000™ system (Radiotherapeutics, Sunnyvale, CA). (**b**) LeVeen™ multitined array electrode

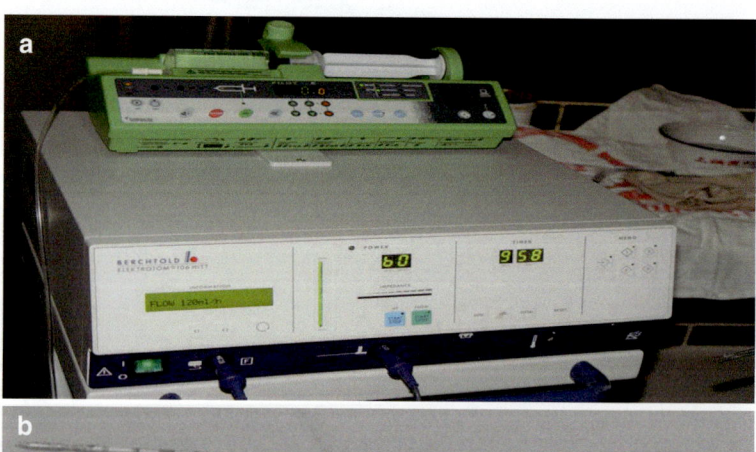

**Fig. 3.5** (**a**) The Elektrotom HiTT® 106 system (Berchtold, Tuttlingen, Germany). (**b**) Monopolar electrode with an active needle tip in 1.5 cm length

nism automatically regulates the heat production in biotissue during saline, maintaining a constant flow. If the impedance exceeds $900 \pm 50$ W, the automated remote control of the syringe pump will release a bolus of 1.2-s duration with the volume of fivefold of nominal flow. For instance, if the continuous saline flow at 40 W is set at 90 mL/h, a bolus of 0.15 mL of saline is infused into tissue. This bolus is permitted only within 5 s in case of increased tissue impedance.

### 3.2.3   CelonPOWER system

Celon*POWER* system is a bipolar RFA system (Celon AG Medical Instruments, OLYMPUS, Japan). The basic concept features two special differences with monopolar devices. Firstly, it is designed as a bipolar unit that does not demand the grounding pads. Both electrodes requiring close to the electrical circuit are located on one application instrument. Secondly, the unit is designed for up to three bipolar electrodes, which are able to operate simultaneously within a single tumor. The general description of how this bipolar system works is illustrated below. For RFA, at least one rigid bipolar coagulation electrode sized 1.8 mm in diameter (15 F) with a 15-cm length shaft (CelonProSurge; Celon AG) is introduced into the tumor. The conducting part of applicators is 40 or 30 mm in length including two electrodes, insulator and tip. In bipolar mode, the high-frequency current transmits between the two electrodes at the tip of the bipolar coagulation electrode and heats up the tissue adjacent the electrodes. An internal liquid circulation of the applicator enables to increase the efficiency of coagulation. The delivery rate is set at 30 mL/min using saline solution at room temperature, and the liquid flow is provided by a triple peristaltic pump in the system. The electrodes are managed by a power control unit at 470 kHz with a maximum output power of 250W (CelonLab Power; Celon AG). The unit can control up to three bipolar electrodes concurrently depending on the actual demands of individual patient in clinical practice. With one of connected bipolar electrode, the unit is in bipolar operating mode. At that time, the device provides an acoustic output for coagulation procedure. If more than one bipolar electrode is connected, the unit is in multi-pin bipolar mode, when all possible electrode pairs are automatically activated with alternating current for up to 2 s based on the actual local tissue resistance. Here, a pair of electrodes not only is defined as the two electrodes located on a specific bipolar applicator shaft but also includes all other possible electrode combinations between the different applicators. Consequently, the current conveys between one electrode of a specific applicator shaft and an electrode at another applicator shaft and passes through the tumor eventually. When three bipolar applicators are placed in a single tumor, there are up to 15 possible combinations (pairs of electrodes) between the current (Fig. 3.6b). If the resistance of an electrode pair increases over threefold of a specific limitation (700 $\Omega$) or the power output is inadequate (less than one-third of the pre-set value), this electrode pair should be discontinued for the next ablation cycle. Power output will be ceased automatically if the resistance of all possible electrode pairs exceeds the threefold limitation, which indicates that dehydration has expanded along with the electrodes completely and the coagulation process has ended. Under microprocessor control, the RF output is divided to each electrode according to the momentary tissue resistance, providing a three-dimensional impedance feedback control [4].

### 3.2.4   Methods to Maximize Ablation Zone

RF electrodes are designed to create an ablative zone with high current density that is large enough to cover the tumor plus coagulative margin. Early electrodes are made of simple bare wires with higher failure rate by water vaporization and tissue dehydration. A work-around is to cool the interior of electrode itself to reduce the temperature at the interface of electrode and tissue. This solution works best when combined with power pulsing. That is, when circuit impedance begins to spike, RF power is suspended for several seconds to equilibrate the tissue temperature and condense

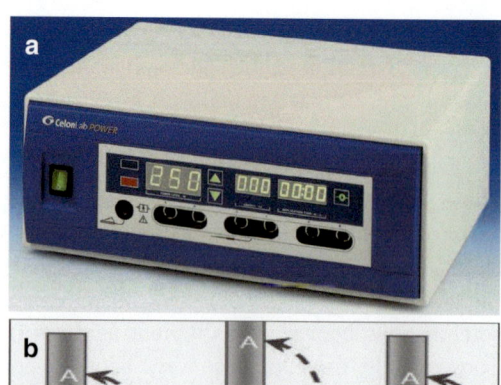

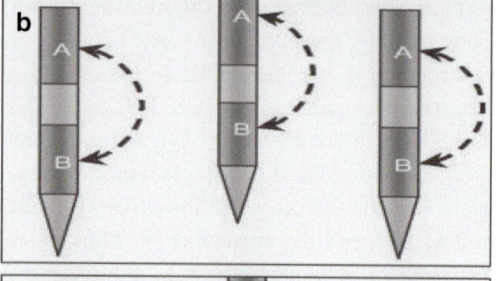

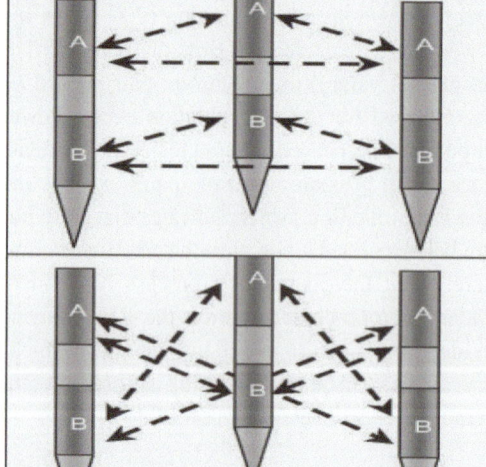

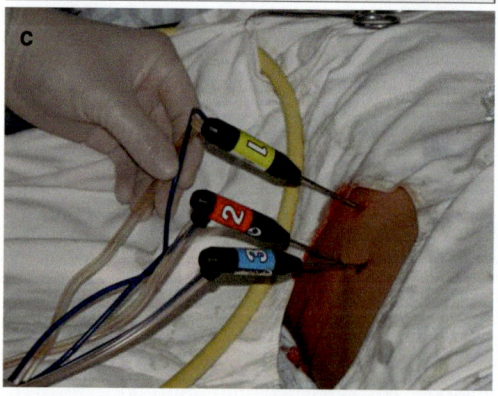

**Fig. 3.6** (**a**) CelonLabPOWER: Bipolar/Multipolar Power Control Unit (RFITT-Generator); (**b**) The principle of three bipolar applicators; (**c**) The application of three bipolar applicators for *CelonLabPOWER* system

the water vapor around the electrodes, which result in the increase of tissue conductivity and thereby allow greater RF power in use during the next heating cycle. Since thermal conduction passing the tissue is much slower than RF heat itself, turning the power off does not detract ablation zone growth. In fact, the combination of electrode cooling and pulsed power can create larger ablation zones than either solution alone.

Another solution to increase the size of RF ablation zone is to spatially distribute the power throughout the tumor volume, either by using multiple-needle electrodes or electrodes with deployable tines. The former solution requires insertion and guidance of up to three electrodes at same time. The electrodes may be operated in parallel as a bipolar array or by sequential switching to improve heating uniformity within the target zone. The latter one only requires the placement of one device, with the umbrella or star-shaped array of deployed tines to provide the necessary distribution of electrical current. These deployable electrodes are larger in diameter than that of cooled electrodes (2.4 mm versus 1.5 mm in diameter). Its tines are difficult to advance into many tumors. Both multiple-electrode and deployable techniques have been shown to increase the size of RF ablations.

It is also possible to augment the electrical conductivity in the medium of surrounding tissue by infusing an ionic fluid such as saline. This technique is beneficial to cool the tissue around the electrode and counteract the low conductivity of dehydrated or charred tissue. This is particularly useful during bipolar RF ablation since the electrode–tissue interface and current path are relatively smaller compared with unipolar ablation with dispersive electrodes. The technique of saline infusion is not popularly used currently due to unpredictable and inhomogenous distribution of infused saline. Some reports have shown that the saline can flow into the body cavity and cause severe heating injury distant to the intended area [14–16].

## Conclusion

Overall, RF ablation has demonstrated the greatest utility in treatment of small tumors (size up to 3 cm in diameter). The application of deployable devices or multiple-electrode systems has intensified the efficacy of RF ablation for medium size tumors (lesion up to 5 cm in diameter) [3, 15]. However, RF ablation still occupies the disadvantages of slow heat generation relatively. A possible solution is to use generator with higher power (up to 1000 W). Nevertheless, such system has not been deployed clinically. Even if higher power is adopted, RF is still limited in use owing to the reliance on electrical current conduction. High-impedance tissue including the RF ablation zone itself precludes the effective RF ablation when insufficient potency is applied. Therefore, investigations at present have been focused on the alternatives of RF for thermal tumor ablation.

## References

1. Llovet JM, Bruix J. Novel advancements in the management of hepatocellular carcinoma in 2008. J Hepatol. 2008;48 Suppl 1:S20–37.
2. Kudo M, Izumi N, Kokudo N, Matsui O, Sakamoto M, et al. Management of hepatocellular carcinoma in Japan: consensus-based clinical practice guidelines proposed by the Japan Society of Hepatology (JSH) 2010 updated version. Dig Dis. 2010;2011(29):339–64.
3. Lau WY, Leung TW, Yu SC, et al. Percutaneous local ablative therapy for hepatocellular carcinoma: a review and look into the future. Ann Surg. 2003;237:171–9.
4. Peng Z-W, Liang H-H, Chen M-S, Zhang Y-J, Li P, Pang X-H, Li J-Q, Zhang Y-Q, Lau WY. Percutaneous radiofrequency ablation for the treatment of hepatocellular carcinomas in the caudate lobe. Eur J Surg Oncol. 2008;34(2):166–72.
5. Chen MS, Li JQ, Zheng Y, et al. A prospective randomized trial comparing percutaneous local ablative therapy and partial hepatectomy for small hepatocellular carcinoma. Ann Surg. 2006;243(3):321–8.
6. Buscarini L, Buscarini E, Di Stasi M, et al. Percutaneous radiofrequency ablation of small hepatocellular carcinoma: long-term results. Eur Radiol. 2001;11(6):914–21.
7. Lencioni R, Crocetti L, Cioni D, et al. Percutaneous radiofrequency ablation of hepatic colorectal metastases. Technique, indications, results, and new promises. Invest Radiol. 2004;39:689–97.
8. Rossi S, Di Stasi M, Buscarini E. Percutaneous RF interstitial thermal ablation in the treatment of hepatic cancer [J]. AJR Am J Roentgenol. 1996;167(3):759–68.
9. Peng Z-W, Zhang Y-J, Chen M-S, Liang H-H, Li J-Q, Zhang Y-Q, Lau WY. Risk factors of survival after percutaneous radiofrequency ablation of hepatocellular carcinoma. Surg Oncol. 2008;17:23–31.
10. Livraghi T, Lazzaroni S, Meloni F. Radiofrequency ablation of hepatocellular carcinoma [J]. Eur J Ultrasound. 2001;13(2):159–66.
11. Brieger J, Pereira PL, Trübenbach J, Schenk M, Kröber SM, Schmidt D, Aubé C, Claussen CD, Schick F. In vivo efficiency of four commercial monopolar radiofrequency ablation systems: a comparative experimental study in pig liver. Invest Radiol. 2003;38(10):609–16.
12. Schmidt D, Trübenbach J, Brieger J, Koenig C, Putzhammer H, Duda SH, Claussen CD, Pereira PL. Automated saline-enhanced radiofrequency thermal ablation: initial results in ex vivo bovine livers. AJR Am J Roentgenol. 2003;180(1):163–5.
13. Pereira PL, Trübenbach J, Schenk M, Subke J, Kroeber S, Schaefer I, Remy CT, Schmidt D, Brieger J, Claussen CD. Radiofrequency ablation: in vivo comparison of four commercially available devices in pig livers. Radiology. 2004;232(2):482–90.
14. Brace C. Thermal tumor ablation in clinical use. IEEE Pulse. 2011;2(5):28–38.
15. Livraghi T, Solbiati L, Meloni MF, et al. Treatment of liver tumors with percutaneous radio-frequency ablation: complications encountered in a multicenter study [J]. Radiology. 2003;226(2):441–51.
16. Zhang YJ, Liang HH, Chen MS, et al. Hepatocellular carcinoma treated with radiofrequency ablation with or without ethanol injection: a prospective randomized trial. Radiology. 2007;244:599–607.

# Initial Clinical Assessment and Patient Selection

# 4

Stephanie H.Y. Lau, Wan Yee Lau, and Eric C.H. Lai

## 4.1 Introduction

For many years, partial hepatectomy and liver transplantation have been considered as the only forms of curative treatment for hepatocellular carcinoma (HCC). Unfortunately, only 10–20 % of HCC is resectable. Anatomic location, size or number of lesions, inadequate liver remnant, or comorbid conditions preclude surgery in the majority of patients. Orthotopic liver transplantation can cure some patients with poor liver function due to underlying cirrhosis, but few patients are eligible because of advanced stage of HCC at initial diagnosis and because of scarcity of liver donors, especially in some parts of the world. Currently, radiofrequency ablation (RFA) is commonly used in patients with small HCC confined to the liver, especially when the tumors are unresectable because of poor general condition of the patients or because of compromised liver func-

tion. Using RFA as a bridge to liver transplantation results in low treatment morbidity and favorable HCC responses and reduces drop-out rate of patients while on the liver transplant waiting list due to HCC progression. Local ablative therapy now competes with partial hepatectomy and liver transplantation as the primary treatment for patients with small HCC. The application of RFA has a number of potential advantages in patients with HCC. The procedure is relatively safe and well tolerated, and its complication rates in most reported series are low. Data have accumulated to support the safety and effectiveness of RFA in selected patients. To achieve good treatment outcomes, proper clinical assessment and patient selection are important. This chapter introduces the clinical assessment and patient selection for RFA [1].

## 4.2 Current Indications for RFA

1. First-line curative treatment for patients with small HCC of less than 5 cm, preferably less than or equal to 3 cm who are not candidates for liver resection or liver transplantation
2. Bridging therapy before liver transplantation
3. Alternative curative treatment to surgery for resectable or transplantable HCC less than or equal to 5 cm, or less than three tumors with each tumor less than 3 cm

S.H.Y. Lau, MBChB(CUHK), MRCS(Ed), FRCS(Ed)
Department of Surgery, Queen Elizabeth Hospital, Hong Kong SAR, China

W.Y. Lau, MD, DSc, FACS, FRCS, FRACS(Hon) (✉)
Chinese Academy of Sciences, Faculty of Medicine, The Chinese University of Hong Kong, Shatin, New Territories, Hong Kong SAR, China
e-mail: josephlau@surgery.cuhk.edu.hk

E.C.H. Lai, MBChB(CUHK), MRCS(Ed), FRACS
Department of Surgery, Pamela Youde Nethersole Eastern Hospital, Hong Kong SAR, China

© Springer Science+Business Media Dordrecht 2016
M. Chen et al. (eds.), *Radiofrequency Ablation for Small Hepatocellular Carcinoma*,
DOI 10.1007/978-94-017-7258-7_4

4. Treatment of recurrent and unresectable HCC
5. Supplementary procedure to liver resection in patients with multiple or bilobar HCC
6. Palliative treatment to control intrahepatic disease
7. Form of treatment in a patient receiving multidisciplinary approach treatment to enhance the effects of local regional (e.g., transcatheter arterial chemoembolization) or systemic treatment (e.g., sorafenib or systemic chemotherapy)

## 4.3 Clinical Assessment

RFA can be carried out percutaneously, laparoscopically, or at open surgery. The laparoscopic and open approaches increase the chance of detection of unknown intrahepatic and extrahepatic tumors, as they allow complete abdominal exploration and intraoperative ultrasonic assessment. The additional advantages of open and laparoscopic approaches are accurate placement of electrodes and possible treatment of tumors in percutaneously inaccessible regions of the liver and tumors in close proximity to or invading adjacent organs. The move from open to laparoscopic to percutaneous techniques loses the advantages of the open but gains the advantages of the minimal invasive approach. Tumor size, number of tumors, site of tumors, liver functional reserve, and general condition of patients are also important considerations in the choice of the RFA approach. Absolute contraindications to RFA are uncorrectable coagulability, extensive ascites not correctable with medication, extensive venous tumor thrombi, and poor associated medical condition, which renders the patient not suitable for any form of sedation or anesthesia. The relative contraindications to RFA are poor liver functional reserve and large HCCs. RFA can still be considered in patients with extrahepatic metastasis or with multiple bilobar HCC if the treatment aims at palliation, especially in patients who receive multidisciplinary treatment for HCC. Therefore, a thorough medical history taking, clinical examination, laboratory investigations, and imaging assessment must be performed on a patient to plan for RFA. Particular attention

should be paid to check whether the patients are taking any anti-platelet or anti-coagulation drugs. All anti-platelet drugs should be stopped at least 1 week before RFA, and warfarin should be converted to heparin before RFA treatment. All underlying medical diseases should be put under control, and any forms of ascites should be controlled with diuretics. Alcohol should be stopped, and patients with hepatitis-B-related hepatitis should have their HBV-DNA checked. It is our belief that patients who are hepatitis B antigen positive should receive antiviral treatment before RFA. Prophylactic antibiotics are commonly given. It is especially indicated in patients with heart valve disease or who has a cardiac/neurological/surgical implant. Thus, a history of drug sensitivity is also important to determine the appropriate prophylactic antibiotic regimen.

The following laboratory tests should be carried out routinely prior to RFA:

1. Complete blood count for hemoglobin, platelet count, and white cell count
2. Coagulation tests including prothrombin time and partial prothrombin time
3. Renal and liver function tests
4. Tumor markers including at least alpha fetoprotein
5. Chest X-ray or cardiopulmonary assessment, if indicated
6. Ultrasonography (USG) and three-phase contrast-enhanced multi-slice helical computed tomography (CT) or dynamic gadolinium-enhanced magnetic resonance imaging (MRI) scan
7. In endemic regions, hepatitis B and C serology

### 4.3.1 Preoperative Imaging and Laboratory Investigations

Ultrasonography is the most popular noninvasive diagnostic imaging technique for patients with HCC. However, its sensitivity in detecting small HCC nodules is variable, and it depends on the experience of the radiologist and the quality of the ultrasonic machine. Intravenous contrast CT or MRI gives better results. Arterial hypervascularity and wash out in the early or delayed venous phases typically denote HCC on CT or MRI. The choice between CT and MRI for diagnosis depends on local expertise and availability. For treatment of HCC with RFA under imaging guidance, USG guidance is most commonly used as it gives real-time imaging of the whole procedure. Although a multimodality fusion imaging system is available, which allows side-by-side display, real-time USG images synchronized with the cross-sectional images of multiphase reconstruction of CT or MRI, thus allowing RFA to be carried out for small HCC nodules which are difficult to detect on conventional USG. This system is available in very few centers [2]. Although AFP concentration is normal (10–20 ng/mL) in some patients with HCC at diagnoses, it is still commonly used as an adjunct to diagnosis of HCC. It is generally accepted that a serum concentration greater than 400 ng/mL in a high-risk patient is diagnostic of HCC. Percutaneous fine-needle biopsy may only be indicated in the setting of inconclusive imaging [3].

The Child-Turcotte-Pugh score is the most common measure to assess liver function before RFA. By staging patients' clinical (presence of ascites and encephalopathy) and laboratory abnormalities (serum albumin, bilirubin, prothrombin time), a score is estimated categorizing patients into three grades of liver dysfunction (Childe-Turcotte-Pugh class A, B, C). Evidence of portal hypertension such as esophagogastric varices, splenomegaly, and thrombocytopenia is also used to assess the liver function. More specific liver function tests may be needed if partial hepatectomy is also needed to be considered during treatment. The most commonly used test in the East is indocyanine green retention at 15 min (ICG-R15).

## 4.3.2 Size of Tumor

RFA is used percutaneously in the large majority of cases, but its application is greatly limited by tumor size and location. Tumor size is of utmost importance to predict outcomes of RFA. An important factor that affects success of RFA is the ability to ablate all viable tumor tissues with an adequate tumor-free margin. In the meta-analysis by Mulier et al., of 5224 treated liver tumors,

local recurrence (meaning, cancer recurrence at the treated site) after percutaneous RFA was 16.9 % in tumors of <3 cm, but it increased to 25.9 % in tumors 3–5 cm and 60 % in tumors >5 cm in size. On the other hand, local recurrence after laparoscopic/open RFA was 3.6 % in tumors of <3 cm but increased to 21.7 % in tumors 3–5 cm and 50 % in tumors >5 cm in size [4]. In the cohort study by Livraghi et al., 218 patients with a single resectable HCC $\leq 2$ cm underwent RFA. After a median follow-up of 31 months, sustained complete response was observed in 216 patients (97.2 %) [5]. Thus, the most suitable size of HCC for RFA should not exceed 3 cm in its longest axis to ensure complete ablation with most of the currently available devices. Recent advances in technique have resulted in larger volumes of tissue ablation, and this may translate into a better ability to treat larger lesions.

## 4.3.3 Number of Tumors

There is no clear cutoff for the number of tumors that can be ablated in a single treatment session. The most important consideration is whether the tumors can be completely ablated within a reasonable time using a reasonable number of sessions of RFA. The greater the number of HCC nodules, the worse are the long-term survival results after RFA treatment. Three is the number that most clinicians would adopt to treat HCC with RFA in a single session.

## 4.3.4 Tumor Location

Pretreatment imaging must also carefully define the location of each lesion with respect to the surrounding structures. A "difficult-to-treat" tumor is generally defined as a tumor located within 1 cm of a vital structure, such as the gastrointestinal tract, gallbladder, diaphragm, major intrahepatic bile ducts or vessels (particularly vessels >3 mm in diameter). Thermal ablation of superficial lesions that are adjacent to any part of the gastrointestinal tract must be avoided because of the risk of thermal injury to gastric or bowel wall.

Laparoscopic or open approach, or the use of special techniques such as intraperitoneal creation of artificial ascites to displace the bowel, can be considered in such cases. If the tumor is close to the gallbladder, cholecystectomy should be considered.

In contrast, thermal ablation of lesions adjacent to large intrahepatic vessels is possible, since flowing blood protects the vascular wall from thermal injury. In these cases, however, the risk of incomplete treatment of neoplastic tissues close to the vessel is increased because of heat sink effect caused by heat loss by convection. In the meta-analysis by Mulier et al., vascular proximity or tumors close to major vascular structures had a recurrence rate of 36.5 %, when compared to 6.3 % for those that were not [5]. A possible solution is to inject ethanol to the tumor tissues adjacent to the vessels before RFA to decrease the chance of inadequate thermal ablation.

Subcapsular tumor location is considered a contraindication to RFA for HCC by some clinicians [6, 7]. However, other clinicians do not exclude subcapsular HCC from RFA [8–12]. The use of RFA with USG guidance is known to be limited in treating subcapsular tumors owing to suboptimal conspicuity of tumor, inadequate electrode path, potential collateral thermal damage, tumor seeding along the needle track, or drop metastasis from subcapsular HCC, resulting in higher complication and local recurrence rates. So far, there have been limited data on the results of RFA for subcapsular HCCs, and the existing data and conclusions are conflicting. Those studies showing inferior results were mainly reported in the early development period of RFA. Recently, there have been more studies showing similar morbidity rates and tumor seeding rates between subcapsular and non-subcapsular tumors after RFA. The role of RFA for subcapsular HCCs remains an issue to be resolved with further studies. The impact of using different approaches to treat these tumors is not well studied too.

## Conclusion

Careful patient selection and selection of the best approach for RFA (percutaneous,

laparoscopy, or laparotomy) will help to minimize procedure-related morbidity and improve oncological outcomes.

## References

1. Lau WY, Lai EC. The current role of radiofrequency ablation in the management of hepatocellular carcinoma: a systematic review. Ann Surg. 2009;249(1):20–5.
2. Makino Y, Imai Y, Igura T, Ohama H, Kogita S, Sawai Y, Fukuda K, Ohashi H, Murakami T. Usefulness of the multimodality fusion imaging on the diagnosis and treatment of hepatocellular carcinoma. Dig Dis. 2012;30(6):580–7.
3. Lau WY, Lai EC. Hepatocellular carcinoma: current management and recent advances. Hepatobiliary Pancreat Dis Int. 2008;7(3):237–57.
4. Mulier S, Ni Y, Jamart J, Ruers T, Marchal G, Michel L. Local recurrence after hepatic radiofrequency coagulation: multivariate meta-analysis and review of contributing factors. Ann Surg. 2005;242:158–71.
5. Livraghi T, Meloni F, Di Stasi M, Rolle E, Solbiati L, Tinelli C, Rossi S. Sustained complete response and complications rates after radiofrequency ablation of very early hepatocellular carcinoma in cirrhosis: Is resection still the treatment of choice? Hepatology. 2008;47(1):82–9.
6. Llovet JM, Vilana R, Brú C, Bianchi L, Salmeron JM, Boix L, Ganau S, Sala M, Pagès M, Ayuso C, Solé M, Rodés J, Bruix J. Barcelona Clínic Liver Cancer (BCLC) Group. Increased risk of tumor seeding after percutaneous radiofrequency ablation for single hepatocellular carcinoma. Hepatology. 2001;33:1124–9.
7. Bonny C, Abergel A, Gayard P, Chouzet S, Ughetto S, Slim K, Rosenfeld L, Guillon R, Poincloux L, Bommelaer G. Radiofrequency ablation of hepatocellular carcinoma in patients with cirrhosis. Gastroenterol Clin Biol. 2002;26(8–9):735–41.
8. Poon RT, Ng KK, Lam CM, Ai V, Yuen J, Fan ST. Radiofrequency ablation for subcapsular hepatocellular carcinoma. Ann Surg Oncol. 2004;11:281–9.
9. Livraghi T, Lazzaroni S, Meloni F, Solbiati L. Risk of tumor seeding after percutaneous radiofrequency ablation for hepatocellular carcinoma. Br J Surg. 2005;92(7):856–8.
10. Shiozawa K, Watanabe M, Wakui N, Ikehara T, Iida K, Sumino Y. Analysis of patients with tumor seeding after percutaneous radiofrequency ablation of hepatocellular carcinoma. Mol Med Rep. 2008;1:851–5.
11. Filippousis P, Sotiropoulou E, Manataki A, Konstantinopoulos O, Thanos L. Radiofrequency ablation of subcapsular hepatocellular carcinoma: single center experience. Eur J Radiol. 2011;77:299–304.
12. Kim JH, Kim PN, Won HJ, Shin YM. Percutaneous radiofrequency ablation using internally cooled wet electrodes for the treatment of hepatocellular carcinoma. AJR Am J Roentgenol. 2012;198:471–6.

# Percutaneous Radiofrequency Thermal Ablation

Zhongguo Zhou and Minshan Chen

## 5.1 Modalities of Imaging-Guided Radiofrequency Thermal Ablation (RFA)

Radiofrequency thermal ablation (RFA) can be performed under the guidance of ultrasound (Fig. 5.1a), computed tomography (CT, Fig. 5.1b), and magnetic resonance imaging (MRI). Ultrasound-guided therapy is the most effectual modality of percutaneous RFA because of adequate targeting capability. However, RFA-generated echogenic cloud of steam during procedure can obscure the target and induce the repositioning of ablation probe and result in overlapping burns difficult. The application of ultrasound contrast available in Europe and Asia is very helpful for ablation operation. Although CT provides the improved depiction of both curative target and RAF ablation probe, working on a gantry is time consuming and less suitable for complex access angles. It is difficult to fit the ablation probes with the gantry, particularly in the treatment of shallow tumors. CT and ultrasound can be used simultaneously to combine the advantages of both of these techniques. Alternatively, image fusion software can be used to superimpose the superior depiction of diagnostic CT and MRI datasets on real-time ultrasound scans to allow the ultrasound-guided probe being placed into sonically occult tumors [1]. MRI guidance, if available, can afford the added advantage of real-time thermal monitoring of the ablation zone.

## 5.2 Patient Evaluation

The joint expertise of an interdisciplinary oncology team involving hepatology, radiation therapy, medical oncology, oncologic surgery, transplant surgery, pathology, radiology, and interventional oncology is critical in the formulation of treatment protocol for patients with malignant tumors. Given the wide range of participants involved, multidisciplinary meetings are useful to triage challenging and complex patients and establish a two-way referral pattern. A typical clinical evaluation includes the history of present illness (HPI), review of systems, medical and surgical experience, performance status, family and social conditions, allergies, medications, physical examination, laboratory tests, imaging comments, and intention of therapeutic options and prognosis, etc.

The documents on previous radiation therapy and chemotherapy, overall course of the disease, and its progression should be particularly noticed in HPL. Performance status is an indicator of entire practical functional level and the self-care ability of patients, which serves as an

Z. Zhou, MD, PhD • M. Chen, MD, PhD (✉)
Department of Hepatobiliary Surgery, Sun Yat-sen University Cancer Center, Guangzhou, China
e-mail: chminsh@mail.sysu.edu.cn

© Springer Science+Business Media Dordrecht 2016
M. Chen et al. (eds.), *Radiofrequency Ablation for Small Hepatocellular Carcinoma*,
DOI 10.1007/978-94-017-7258-7_5

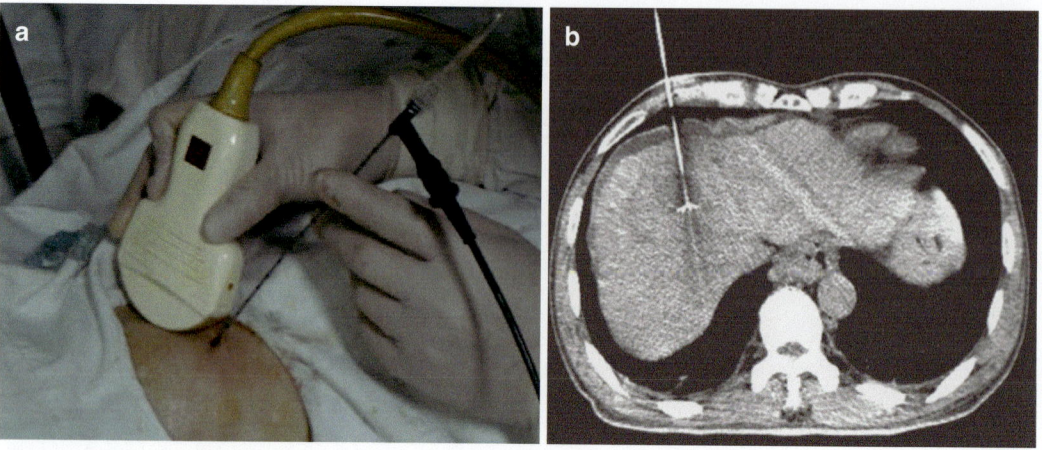

**Fig. 5.1** RFA performed under the guidance of ultrasound (**a**) and CT (**b**)

index of patients' well being and is one of the most powerful indexes of prognosis for overall survival rate. The Eastern Cooperative Oncology Group Scale of Performance Status is a 6-point scale ranging from 0 to 5. Point 0 represents that the patient has normal activities without limitation, and point 5 indicates the death of a patient [2]. Evaluation of health-related quality of life in patients is somewhat similar to the estimation of performance status; however, performance status seems more directly focused on the ability of patients to perform daily life activities (eating, bathing, dressing) and other activities (driving, shopping, paying bills) [3]. The laboratory tests should include a complete blood count, creatinine concentration, prothrombin time, and/or international normalized ratio. Additional tests such as a liver function panel, relevant tumor markers such as α-fetoprotein, carcinoembryonic antigen, chromogranin A, and CA199 should be assayed for identifying specific undetermined malignancy. Personal review of cross-sectional imaging is critical during the process of evaluation; simply reading the radiological report is a far way to achieve satisfaction. Baseline imaging should be taken optimally within a month prior to therapy, which will be used for comparisons of tumor curative response more accurately later. Careful evaluation of tumor number, size, morphology, adjacent structures, and extrahepatic metastases will benefit the selection of treatment modality and feasibility.

The prognosis of patient is closely associated with tumor staging. The Child-Turcotte-Pugh (CTP) score is implemented for assessment of liver disease, which is not a tumor staging system but rather a measure of hepatic reserve. The CTP score is derived from a point system based on serum levels of albumin, total bilirubin, prothrombin time, the presence of ascites, and hepatic encephalopathy. While the CTP score increases, surgical risk increases as well and the life expectancy decreases correspondingly. The HCC staging systems are composed of the Okuda staging system, the Cancer of the Liver Italian Program classification (CLIP), the Barcelona Clinic Liver Cancer Staging classification (BCLC), the United Network for Organ Sharing (UNOS TNM), the Chinese University Prognostic Index, the Liver Cancer Study Group of Japan, and the American Joint Committee on Cancer/International Union Against Cancer. No single staging system has been proven better than the other. Nevertheless, the BCLC and CLIP staging systems of HCC appear to be the more preferred systems for interventional oncologists. Currently, a variety of transplant centers use the UNOS staging in clinical practice [4].

After a comprehensive evaluation, all therapeutic options should be considered when formulating a treatment regimen. Orthotopic liver transplant is a curative option for a part of HCC patients. Surgical resection of HCC is often not an option due to inadequate functional liver reserve (FLR) of cirrhosis [4]. Interventional oncologists play a key role in the management of patients who are not eligible or who are unwilling to accept surgery. Based on the tumor size and tumor number, ablation may be the sole choice of operation; alternatively, it may be combined with other regional and systemic therapies. The location of tumors will affect the feasibility and safety of percutaneous ablation when close to great vessels versus a regular surgical approach (Figs. 5.2, 5.3, 5.4, and 5.5). Such patients are a rich source of two-way referrals with surgical oncology.

## 5.3 Indications and Contraindications of RFA

The Milan criteria (solitary HCC <5 cm in diameter, multiple HCCs ≤3 in number and each tumor < 3 cm in diameter) have been accepted as the indications of RFA in many institutes. The limitation of tumor numbers in patients with multiple HCCs depends on several clinical considerations, including the general performance of the patients, the capacity of tolerance to surgical procedure, the skill and experience of the operator, and the whole processing time. Therefore, the number of tumors treatable in one session should be determined based on the individual situation

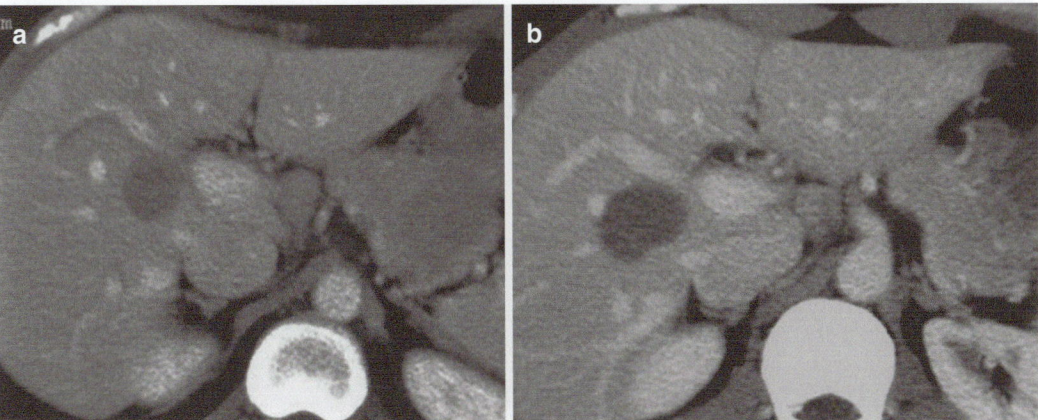

**Fig. 5.2** Tumor's location closed to portal vein. Before RFA (**a**) and after RFA (**b**)

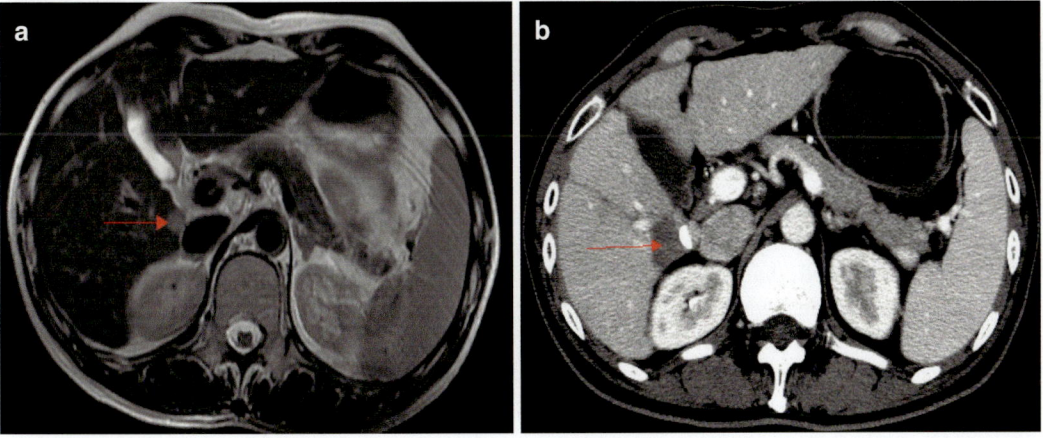

**Fig. 5.3** Tumor's (*arrows*) location closed to inferior vena cava. Before RFA (**a**) and after RFA plus TACE (**b**)

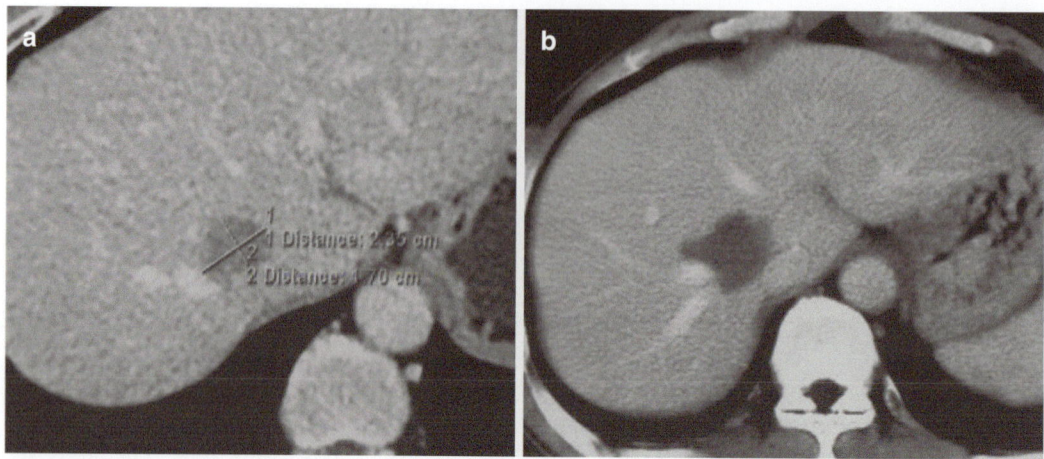

**Fig. 5.4** Tumor's location closed to inferior vena cava and hepatic vein. Before RFA (**a**) and after RFA (**b**)

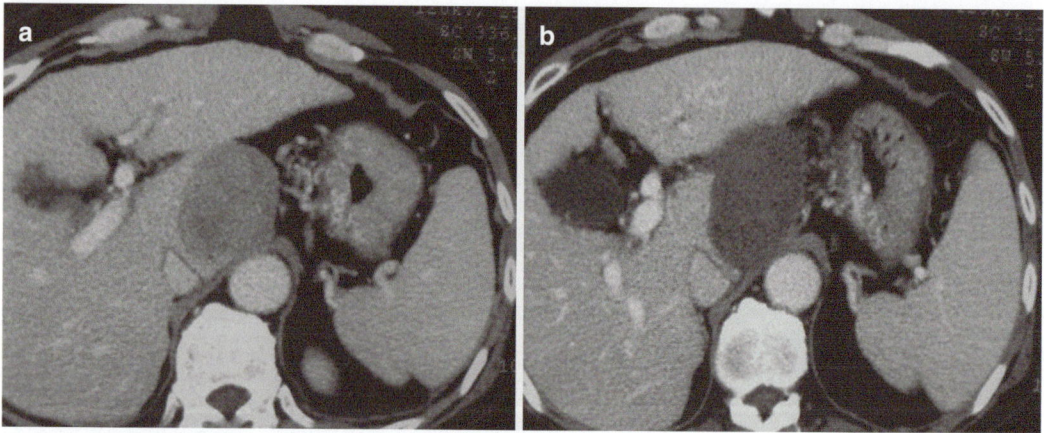

**Fig. 5.5** Tumor in caudate lobe. Before RFA (**a**) and after RFA (**b**)

although "no greater than three" appears to be the most widely accepted criterion.

With respect to the maximal tumor diameter, there are several issues that are required to be taken into consideration. Apparently, RFA has limited capability to completely ablate the tumors with "large size." However, what is the definition of "large size" is undetermined [5, 6]. Some investigators suggested that the borderline of HCC <2 cm in diameter was considered "large size," which was used as a criterion for patients who received RFA at a very early tumor stage in the Barcelona Clinic Liver Cancer (BCLC) staging system and showed excellent long-term outcomes after RFA treatment. From the histopathological perspective, HCC <2 cm in diameter is known to have a greater well-differentiated area and fewer microsatellite lesions (3 % of the cases), which are usually within 5 mm of the tumor with less portal microinvasion [7]. The treatment guidelines published by the BCLC group in 2012 recommended that ablation prior to small HCCs resection is a curative option to patients, except liver transplantation [8], which is a major revision from the previous version. Given these facts, we propose that RFA can be used as a first-line therapy for patients with a small HCC <2 cm in diameter, even if the tumor resection is a feasible surgical option.

In view of the inadequacy of RFA devices available currently and the disadvantages of overlapping ablation techniques and the ablative margin, the patients with HCC sized ≥5.0 cm in diameter should not be treated with RFA alone [8]. For them, other therapeutic options or combination therapy should be considered.

Nonetheless, what about the patients who are in gray zone between these situations? It is evident that the larger tumor size is commonly accompanied by a higher incidence of local tumor progression (LTP) after RFA, whereas a larger ablation zone would increase the risks of complications. Therefore, the decision of whether to take RFA for HCCs patients in gray zone should be made only after serious evaluation of hepatic functional reserve of the patients and the availability of other therapeutic modalities. This is even more important if we take into account that extending the tumor size to 3 cm in diameter increases the chance of spreading satellite nodules to 19 % [9]. RFA should be avoided in cases of impending portal venous invasion or in patients with risk factors for possible diffuse recurrence [10]. When tumor resection is infeasible and RFA is replaced for HCC patients in gray zone, skill to enlarge the ablation area or combination therapy such as TACE should be adopted. The survival benefits of combination therapy of RFA plus TACE superior to RFA alone in the treatment of HCCs sized at 3–5 cm in diameter were demonstrated in a randomized controlled trial (RCT) [11]. A consensus-based clinical practice manual [12] of the Japanese Society of Hepatology recommends to taking RFA combined with TACE in the management of HCC with size larger than 3 cm.

As for hepatic functions, it should be minimally kept at the level which is able to tolerate the loss of hepatic parenchyma induced by ablation in order to benefit from the tumor removal in terms of survival gain. Thus, patients with Child-Pugh class C are not usually indicated for RFA. Contraindications of percutaneous RFA include uncorrectable coagulopathy, liver failure, unadjustable proximity to critical structures, and extrahepatic metastases (except small, slow-growing lung metastases or minimal adenopathy) [13]. Mortality of HCC during the treatment ranged from 0.1 % to 0.5%, and the incidences of major complication were from 2.2 % to 3.1%. The most common causes of death were sepsis,

hepatic failure, colon perforation, and portal vein thrombosis except for several patients who died of cardiac or pericardial injury. Tumors in precarious locations should be referred for laparoscopic or open ablation. The most common complications were intraperitoneal bleeding hepatic abscess, bile duct injury, hepatic decompensation, and grounding pad burns. Tract ablation or embolization may help to prevent bleeding. Patients with prior biliary stents or surgery are at increased risk for liver abscess and should receive prophylactic antibiotics [14]. Ablation zones should be kept at 1 cm away from the liver hilum to avoid major bile duct injury. The grounding pads should be checked periodically during the procedure, especially during prolonged ablations at high wattage to avoid skin burns. Tumor seeding metastasis occurred in 0.2–0.6 % of patients and was of particular concern in patients who were candidates for liver transplantation [15].

## 5.4 Percutaneous RFA Procedure

Percutaneous ablation is usually conducted in an outpatient clinic under intravenous moderate sedation or monitored anesthesia care. Ablation with heat is very painful and requires deep sedation to induce the patients with spontaneous breathing but no voice response. An oxygen mask is often required to maintain adequate oxygen saturation. Pay attention to proper neck and jaw position of the patient to maintain an unobstructed airway. Electrocardiogram, blood pressure, pulse, and pulse oximetry should be monitored throughout the procedure. After careful review of the diagnostic images, preliminary scanning is performed to choose an appropriate site for probe entry based on the conditions of trajectory to the target, probe length, nontarget structures, and physical constraints of the CT or MRI gantry. When RFA operation is close to the bowel, abdominal wall, or diaphragm, infusion of 500–1000 mL 5 % dextrose to develop artificial ascites is necessary to protect against thermal injury of nontarget tissues and decrease intra- and post-operative pain [16]. The type and number of probes and the number of ablations depend on the operative goal to achieve a total ablation zone 5–10 mm larger than the tumor entity. This additional circumferential margin of ablation is beneficial to treat the microscopic satellite lesions and mitigates local recurrence. If the tumor diameter is equal to or larger than the ablative size of a single ablation, it requires multiple overlapping burns. Geometric modeling assuming spherical target and ablation zones implicate that eight perfectly overlapped ablations would be needed to initialize an ablative coverage of 1 cm larger than tumor size. An impossibility in clinical practice accounts for the high local failure rate as tumor size larger than 3 cm in diameter. Another technical consideration is perfusion of mediated cooling via adjacent veins (the "heat-sink" effect). Veins even as small as 3 mm have sufficient flow to produce convective cooling in ablation area. Placement of a balloon occlusion catheter into the hepatic vein or inferior vena cava during operation may help to mitigate the burning effect [17]. RFA operation is monitored by automated systems within the generator that provide the feedback of time, temperature, and/or impedance with management resolution specified by an individual manufacturer. The most thermal systems allow to perform ablation procedure along with the needle track to decrease the risk of bleeding and tumor seeding metastasis. Triple-phase enhanced CT or MRI may be applied at the end of the procedure to evaluate the completion of ablation and identify the intense inflammatory reaction to RFA resulting in substantial perilesional enhancement and abnormal perfusion patterns in surrounding liver. The ablation zone shows a nonenhancing area. Peripheral, irregular nodular areas of enhancement near the ablation area are considered of residual tumor.

### 5.4.1    Skill for Larger Ablation Zones

A conventional RF electrode is able to provoke a coagulation necrosis area less than 1.6 cm in diameter maximally [18]. This function will be reduced by tissue vaporization and/or carbonization, acting as an insulator of electrical currents during performance of RFA. In order to avoid this inherent restriction, several adaptations have been accepted for RF devices available currently, including expandable multi-tined designs, internal cooling by chilled saline, clustered design, pulsing of RF energy, and concomitant saline infusion into the tissue. These techniques contribute to enlarging the RFA zone to 3–4 cm. The application of multiple overlapping ablations or multiple electrodes simultaneously can further increase the area of ablation [18]. Taken together into consideration, HCC sized up to 4–5 cm in diameter can now be treated potentially by RAF technique as well, at least in theory.

### 5.4.2    Skill for Accurate Targeting

Another crucial factor to confine the application of RFA is the complexity of accurate targeting in certain situations. US is the most common device for guidance of RFA. US-guided visibility of HCC is hindered by a complicated tumor location with a poor acoustic window, which is more likely to present in a cirrhotic liver, or by the small size tumor in a background of macronodular cirrhosis. In the study of Kim et al. [19], US-guided percutaneous RFA was unfeasible in 33.1 % HCC patients mainly ascribed to undetectable tumor. Currently, several skills have been proposed for overcoming this disadvantage. The technique of infusion fluid into the pleural or peritoneal cavity, namely, artificial pleural effusion or artificial ascites, is useful to clear the acoustic window. Minami et al. [20] reported the effectiveness of artificial pleural effusion in achieving a high rate of complete necrosis of HCC (96.4 %). Rhim et al. [21] reported a similar rate of complete treatment (96.0 %) using artificial ascites skill. The artificial ascites is known to be particularly useful in minimizing or preventing the risk of collateral thermal injury by displacing the bowel loop or the diaphragm away from the RFA zone [22]

Fusion imaging is also a useful tool to overcome poor conspicuity of tumors on conventional US imaging. With this method, volumetric CT or MRI data obtained previously are reformatted on a real-time basis in sync with a B-mode US image with the help of an electromagnetic field generator and a sensor attached to the US transducer. Using this technique, Lee et al. [23] reported a technical success rate of 100 % in the treatment of tiny HCCs (mean diameter, 1.0 cm) in patients who had poor conspicuity in US examination. Song et al. [24] applied this method for HCCs patients who were completely non-visible in planning US examinations and showed that 53.3 % of the patients could be treated by RFA. Contrast-enhanced US examination is also helpful for delineating poorly visible HCC. The old generation of contrast agents (e.g., Levovist [Bayer-Schering Phama, Berlin, Germany] and SonoVue [Bracco, Milan Italy]) could only describe hypervascular HCC at the vascular phase. However, the novel microbubble agent Sonazoid (GE Healthcare, Milwaukee, WI) can additionally depict the tumor at post-vascular phase or Kupffer phase (i.e., 10–15 min after administration) as an echo-void lesion on a background of echorich parenchyma, which is much more sustainable. Consequently, RFA is easier for operation technically. Masuzaki et al. [25] reported a significantly increased detection rate of HCC with Sonazoid-enhanced US than those with conventional US (93.2 % vs. 83.5 %, p = 0.04). Combination of fusion imaging with Sonazoid-enhanced US is able to further improve the detection rate of tumors. Min et al. [26] reported that 92 % of fusion imaging in inconspicuous small HCCs might be feasible for RFA after additional Sonazoid enhancement US examination.

## 5.5    Complications of RFA

There have been substantially more data in terms of the complications occurring in liver ablation than those occurring in any other sites. Overall, the incidence of major complications (2.2–5.7 %) and the mortality (0–1.4 %) were lower in thermal ablation of liver malignancies [27–33]. In contrast, the mortality and major complication rates of microwave ablation (MWA) were reported as 0–0.4 % and 2.6–4.6 %, respectively. In recent studies, the types and incidences of complications

caused by HCC RFA and MWA were similar and comparable in clinical setting [28, 34]. The causes of death involved intestinal perforation, portal vein thrombosis, liver failure, septic shock, and massive hepatic hemorrhage [31, 32, 35]. The major complications included hemorrhage, liver failure, injuries to bowel and biliary tree, infections such as abscesses and peritonitis, vascular thrombosis, hepatic infarction, pleural complications (pneumothorax, hemothorax, large effusion drainage), biliary strictures, bilomas, cholecystitis, bronchobiliary fistulas, arteriovenous fistula leading to rapid tumor dissemination, skin burns, and tumor seeding metastasis.

## References

1. Iida H, Aihara T, Ikuta S, et al. Comparative study of percutaneous radiofrequency ablation and hepatic resection for small, poorly differentiated hepatocellular carcinomas. Hepatol Res. 2014;44:E156–62.
2. Sorensen JB, Klee M, Palshof T, et al. Performance status assessment in cancer patients. An inter-observer variability study. Br J Cancer. 1993;67:773–5.
3. Gomaa AI, Khan SA, Leen EL, et al. Diagnosis of hepatocellular carcinoma. World J Gastroenterol. 2009;15:1301–14.
4. Gervais DA, Goldberg SN, Brown DB, et al. Society of interventional radiology position statement on percutaneous radiofrequency ablation for the treatment of liver tumors. J Vasc Interv Radiol. 2009;20:S342–7.
5. Livraghi T, Meloni F, Di Stasi M, et al. Sustained complete response and complications rates after radiofrequency ablation of very early hepatocellular carcinoma in cirrhosis: is resection still the treatment of choice? Hepatology. 2008;47:82–9.
6. Wang JH, Wang CC, Hung CH, et al. Survival comparison between surgical resection and radiofrequency ablation for patients in BCLC very early/early stage hepatocellular carcinoma. J Hepatol. 2012;56:412–8.
7. Livraghi T. Single HCC smaller than 2 cm: surgery or ablation: interventional oncologist's perspective. J Hepatobiliary Pancreat Sci. 2010;17:425–9.
8. Forner A, Llovet JM, Bruix J. Hepatocellular carcinoma. Lancet. 2012;379:1245–55.
9. Okusaka T, Okada S, Ueno H, et al. Satellite lesions in patients with small hepatocellular carcinoma with reference to clinicopathologic features. Cancer. 2002;95:1931–7.
10. Lee HY, Rhim H, Lee MW, et al. Early diffuse recurrence of hepatocellular carcinoma after percutaneous radiofrequency ablation: analysis of risk factors. Eur Radiol. 2013;23:190–7.

11. Morimoto M, Numata K, Kondou M, et al. Midterm outcomes in patients with intermediate-sized hepatocellular carcinoma: a randomized controlled trial for determining the efficacy of radiofrequency ablation combined with transcatheter arterial chemoembolization. Cancer. 2010;116:5452–60.

12. Kudo M, Okanoue T. Japan Society of H: Management of hepatocellular carcinoma in Japan: consensus-based clinical practice manual proposed by the Japan Society of Hepatology. Oncology. 2007;72(1):2–15.

13. Woo S, Lee JM, Yoon JH, et al. Small- and medium-sized hepatocellular carcinomas: monopolar radiofrequency ablation with a multiple-electrode switching system-mid-term results. Radiology. 2013; 268:589–600.

14. Elias D, Di Pietroantonio D, Gachot B, et al. Liver abscess after radiofrequency ablation of tumors in patients with a biliary tract procedure. Gastroenterol Clin Biol. 2006;30:823–7.

15. Stigliano R, Marelli L, Yu D, et al. Seeding following percutaneous diagnostic and therapeutic approaches for hepatocellular carcinoma. What is the risk and the outcome? Seeding risk for percutaneous approach of HCC. Cancer Treat Rev. 2007;33:437–47.

16. Hinshaw JL, Laeseke PF, Winter 3rd TC, et al. Radiofrequency ablation of peripheral liver tumors: intraperitoneal 5% dextrose in water decreases postprocedural pain. AJR Am J Roentgenol. 2006; 186:S306–10.

17. de Baere T, Bessoud B, Dromain C, et al. Percutaneous radiofrequency ablation of hepatic tumors during temporary venous occlusion. AJR Am J Roentgenol. 2002;178:53–9.

18. Rhim H, Goldberg SN, Dodd GD 3rd, et al. Essential techniques for successful radio-frequency thermal ablation of malignant hepatic tumors. Radiographics. 2001;(21 Spec No):S17–35; discussion S36–9.

19. Kim JE, Kim YS, Rhim H, et al. Outcomes of patients with hepatocellular carcinoma referred for percutaneous radiofrequency ablation at a tertiary center: analysis focused on the feasibility with the use of ultrasonography guidance. Eur J Radiol. 2011;79: e80–4.

20. Minami Y, Kudo M, Kawasaki T, et al. Percutaneous ultrasound-guided radiofrequency ablation with artificial pleural effusion for hepatocellular carcinoma in the hepatic dome. J Gastroenterol. 2003;38: 1066–70.

21. Rhim H, Lim HK, Kim YS, et al. Percutaneous radiofrequency ablation with artificial ascites for hepatocellular carcinoma in the hepatic dome: initial experience. AJR Am J Roentgenol. 2008;190:91–8.

22. Song I, Rhim H, Lim HK, et al. Percutaneous radiofrequency ablation of hepatocellular carcinoma abutting the diaphragm and gastrointestinal tracts with the use of artificial ascites: safety and technical efficacy in 143 patients. Eur Radiol. 2009;19:2630–40.

23. Lee MW, Rhim H, Cha DI, et al. Percutaneous radiofrequency ablation of hepatocellular carcinoma: fusion imaging guidance for management of lesions with poor conspicuity at conventional sonography. AJR Am J Roentgenol. 2012;198:1438–44.

24. Song KD, Lee MW, Rhim H, et al. Fusion imaging-guided radiofrequency ablation for hepatocellular carcinomas not visible on conventional ultrasound. AJR Am J Roentgenol. 2013;201:1141–7.

25. Masuzaki R, Shiina S, Tateishi R, et al. Utility of contrast-enhanced ultrasonography with Sonazoid in radiofrequency ablation for hepatocellular carcinoma. J Gastroenterol Hepatol. 2011;26:759–64.

26. Min JH, Lim HK, Lim S, et al. Radiofrequency ablation of very-early-stage hepatocellular carcinoma inconspicuous on fusion imaging with B-mode US: value of fusion imaging with contrast-enhanced US. Clin Mol Hepatol. 2014;20:61–70.

27. Liang P, Wang Y, Yu X, et al. Malignant liver tumors: treatment with percutaneous microwave ablation--complications among cohort of 1136 patients. Radiology. 2009;251:933–40.

28. Ding J, Jing X, Liu J, et al. Complications of thermal ablation of hepatic tumours: comparison of radiofrequency and microwave ablative techniques. Clin Radiol. 2013;68:608–15.

29. Buscarini E, Buscarini L. Radiofrequency thermal ablation with expandable needle of focal liver malignancies: complication report. Eur Radiol. 2004;14:31–7.

30. Nemcek AA. Complications of radiofrequency ablation of neoplasms. Semin Intervent Radiol. 2006;23:177–87.

31. Howenstein MJ, Sato KT. Complications of radiofrequency ablation of hepatic, pulmonary, and renal neoplasms. Semin Intervent Radiol. 2010;27:285–95.

32. Takaki H, Yamakado K, Nakatsuka A, et al. Frequency of and risk factors for complications after liver radiofrequency ablation under CT fluoroscopic guidance in 1500 sessions: single-center experience. AJR Am J Roentgenol. 2013;200:658–64.

33. Koda M, Murawaki Y, Hirooka Y, et al. Complications of radiofrequency ablation for hepatocellular carcinoma in a multicenter study: An analysis of 16 346 treated nodules in 13 283 patients. Hepatol Res. 2012;42:1058–64.

34. Bertot LC, Sato M, Tateishi R, et al. Mortality and complication rates of percutaneous ablative techniques for the treatment of liver tumors: a systematic review. Eur Radiol. 2011;21:2584–96.

35. de Baere T, Risse O, Kuoch V, et al. Adverse events during radiofrequency treatment of 582 hepatic tumors. AJR Am J Roentgenol. 2003;181:695–700.

# Laparoscopic and Open RFA

# 6

Eric C.H. Lai, Stephanie H.Y. Lau, and Wan Yee Lau

## 6.1 Introduction

Tumor diameter, number and position, liver function, and general health of a patient must be considered when evaluating radiofrequency ablation (RFA) for hepatocellular carcinoma. There are three primary approaches to RFA: percutaneous, laparoscopic, and open. The main goal in each of the RFA approaches is capability of safely achieving complete tumor ablation with adequate ablation margins. The choice of the different approaches for RFA should be tailored to the individual patient according to the tumor volume and location.

This chapter illustrates the advantages, disadvantages, and role of surgical (laparoscopic and open) RFA.

E.C.H. Lai, MBChB(CUHK), MRCS(Ed), FRACS
Department of Surgery, Pamela Youde Nethersole
Eastern Hospital, Hong Kong SAR, China

S.H.Y. Lau, MBChB(CUHK), MRCS(Ed), FRCS(Ed)
Department of Surgery, Queen Elizabeth Hospital,
Hong Kong SAR, China

W.Y. Lau, MD, DSc, FACS, FRCS, FRACS(Hon) (✉)
Chinese Academy of Sciences, Faculty of Medicine,
The Chinese University of Hong Kong,
Shatin, New Territories, Hong Kong SAR, China
e-mail: josephlau@surgery.cuhk.edu.hk

## 6.2 Advantages and Disadvantages of Different RFA Approaches

The advantages of percutaneous RFA include less invasiveness, reduced postoperative pain, shorter hospitalization, reduced costs, and lower discomfort in repeating the procedure. However, surgical RFA allows better cancer staging, avoidance of adjacent organ injury, accessibility to all liver regions with better application of RFA electrodes in terms of probe direction, and creation of overlapping ablation zones for large tumors. Open RFA also gives the chance to perform simultaneous other organ resection. Its disadvantages are the need for general anesthesia, increased invasiveness, and longer duration of hospital stay [1].

## 6.3 Role of Laparoscopic and Open RFA

In the early developmental period, the use of percutaneous RFA was confined to patients with a few small tumors in the periphery and away from adjacent organs. However, with advancements in technology, difficult lesions can now be treated. For tumors which are close to adjacent organs, surgical RFA is still a safer way to use because adjacent organs can be protected from injury (Figs. 6.1 and 6.2), e.g., the diaphragm or

© Springer Science+Business Media Dordrecht 2016
M. Chen et al. (eds.), *Radiofrequency Ablation for Small Hepatocellular Carcinoma*,
DOI 10.1007/978-94-017-7258-7_6

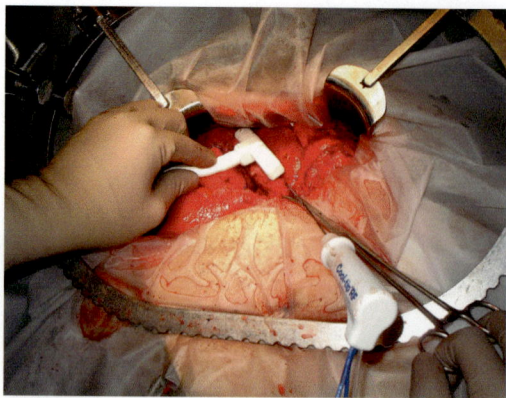

**Fig. 6.1** Open RFA

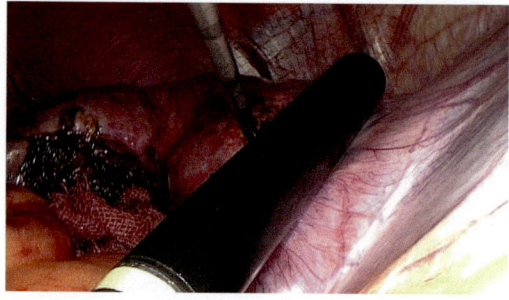

**Fig. 6.2** Laparoscopic RFA

gastrointestinal tract can be protected and displaced away from the ablative sites using soaked normal saline gauze packing or by retractors. However, for tumors which are close to the gallbladder, cholecystectomy is needed in conjunction with the ablation procedure. For subcapsular tumors, percutaneous RFA under ultrasound guidance is known to have its own inherent problems, which include suboptimal conspicuity of tumor, inadequate electrode placement, and potential collateral thermal damage to adjacent tissues. To overcome these problems, RFA using artificial ascites was introduced not only to enhance the sonic window but also to avoid collateral thermal injury by separating the adjacent organs from the tumor. Although this technique has been shown to be feasible and safe in selected patients, the presence of ascites potentially decreases the "tamponade effect" of the opposing parietal abdominal wall against the liver, and the free space introduced by artificial ascites can facilitate dissemination of

viable tumor cells [2–5], thus increasing the risk of peritoneal seeding, and surgical RFA is a better approach under such a situation.

The surgical RFA approach is generally applied to patients with multiple large tumors which range from 3 to 5 cm or which are close to a large vessel. Surgical RFA allows for temporary occlusion of hepatic artery and portal vein, the Pringle's maneuver, which practically stops all blood inflow to the liver. As the cooling effect from the blood inflow is minimized, large tumors are more likely to be completely ablated. It also facilitates bile duct cooling by using an endoscopic nasobiliary drainage (ENBD) tube during RFA for HCC close to major bile ducts. If multiple RFA ablations with overlapping ablation zones are needed for large tumors, surgical RFA is more suitable. If the patient also presents with a separate tumor that cannot undergo RFA but is suitable to be resected, it can be surgically resected during the same operation. Moreover, surgical RFA enables identification and control of bleeding after treatment of superficial tumors and avoidance of seeding along the needle track.

The disadvantages of open RFA are similar to those of other open surgeries, as it is more expensive, requires general anesthesia and longer hospital stay, and is associated with more pain. In addition, as percutaneous RFA technique has improved much in the last decade, open RFA now contributes only to a small proportion of RFA procedures in most centers. As a consequence, there are very limited data on open RFA. One non-randomized study showed percutaneous RFA to have a significantly shorter hospital stay (4.1 vs. 7.6 days) and a lower morbidity rate (2.3 % vs. 8.8 %) than open RFA [6].

Laparoscopic RFA is currently more commonly adopted than open RFA. Laparoscopic RFA combines many of the benefits of both the percutaneous and open approaches. However, a history of previous abdominal surgery with significant intraabdominal adhesions may preclude the use of the laparoscopic approach. Laparoscopic RFA is a safe treatment for liver tumors in deep locations, as well as superficial nodules adjacent to the diaphragm and organs, or for multiple lesions. The complication and mortality rates have been reported to range from 3.2 % to 27 % and from 0 % to 1.9 %, respectively [7–11]. Three non-randomized comparative studies consistently showed that laparoscopic RFA had significantly lower intraoperative blood loss, shorter operative time, and shorter postoperative hospital stay, when compared with open RFA [12–14]. In addition, laparoscopic intraoperative ultrasound during laparoscopic RFA allows a much more accurate staging than preoperative imagings. Laparoscopic intraoperative ultrasound has been reported with great accuracy during the procedure, permitting to detect 13.3–46.1 % new HCC nodules missed at preoperative imagings [15–18]. The laparoscopic approach also has the advantages of the open approach, such as applying the Pringle's Maneuver, or to carry out concomitant resectional procedures. However, it is technically more challenging. For those tumors which are close to the dome of the liver or when the right posterior sector is shrunken in cirrhotic liver, the degree of freedom for introduction of the RFA electrodes is less than with open RFA. In expert centers, these tumors in such difficult locations can still be treated by laparoscopic RFA. In the series of caudate lobe HCC treated by laparoscopic RFA reported by the Chinese PLA General Hospital in Beijing, 27 patients underwent laparoscopic caudate lobe RFA for solitary small HCC with a mean tumor size of 2.8 cm [19]. The 1-, 3-, and 5-year overall survival rates were 96.3, 74.1, and 62.9 %, respectively. The 1-, 3-, and 5-year disease-free survival rates after RFA were 92.6, 44.4 and 33.3 %, respectively. The most common postoperative complication in that series was pleural effusion (25.9 %), followed by transient hemoglobinuria (7.4 %). For oncological outcomes, most reported series were on patients with unresectable small HCC. After a mean follow-up of 14.3–36.9 months, 2.9–69.5 % showed local recurrences; 4.8–22.3 %, remote recurrences; and <2 %, both local and remote recurrences [20–24]. Based on the limited evidence, there were no significant differences in the overall survival, recurrence-free survival, and local recurrence rates between the laparoscopic RFA group and the open RFA group. There have been more recent studies comparing liver resection with laparoscopic RFA for small HCC. Four non-randomized studies showed longer duration of hospital stay and higher rates of postoperative complications in the liver resection group [25–28]. However, the oncological outcomes were conflicting. Karabulut et al. showed no significant difference in disease-free survival between the RFA group (median tumor size, 3.1 cm) and the resection group (median tumor size, 5.3 cm), but the 5-year actual survival was significantly higher (40 % vs. 21 %) in the resection group [25]. Santambrogio et al. showed similar 5-year actuarial survival rates (54 % vs. 41 %) after resection (mean tumor size, 2.91 cm) and after RFA (mean tumor size, 2.66 cm) for solitary HCC with Child-Pugh class A liver cirrhosis, despite a marked increase in HCC recurrence rates after RFA (6 % vs. 24 %) [26]. Lai et al. showed significantly lower 5-year disease-free survival (40 % vs. 60 %) in the RFA group (mean tumor size, 1.8 cm) than in the resection group (mean tumor size, 2.9 cm) but similar 5-year overall survivals in the two groups (84 % vs. 71 %) [27]. Tohmeno et al. showed no significant differences in 5-year overall survival (35 % vs. 47 %) and 5-year disease-free survival (28 % vs. 34 %) between the RFA group (mean tumor size, 2.36 cm) and the resection group (mean tumor size, 3.07 cm) [28].

In general, surgical RFA should be considered if any of the following conditions are present: (a) significant coagulopathy, (b) large tumors (but <5 cm) or multiple lesions requiring repeated punctures, (c) superficial lesions adjacent to visceral structures, (d) lesions with a very difficult or impossible percutaneous approach, (e) short interval of recurrence of HCC following percutaneous RFA. Currently, there is no evidence which comes from randomized trial comparing percutaneous RFA and surgical RFA. All the evidence were based on cohort studies and non-randomized retrospective studies.

## Conclusion

Careful patient selection and use of the best approach (percutaneous, laparoscopy, or laparotomy) help to minimize complications after RFA. The choice of the different approaches of RFA should be tailored to the individual patients according to tumor volume and location.

# References

1. Lau WY, Lai EC. The current role of radiofrequency ablation in the management of hepatocellular carcinoma: a systematic review. Ann Surg. 2009;249(1):20–5.
2. Kondo Y, Yoshida H, Shiina S, Tateishi R, Teratani T, Omata M. Artificial ascites technique for percutaneous radiofrequency ablation of liver cancer adjacent to the gastrointestinal tract. Br J Surg. 2006;93(10):1277–82.
3. Sartori S, Tombesi P, Macario F, Nielsen I, Tassinari D, Catellani M, Abbasciano V. Subcapsular liver tumors treated with percutaneous radiofrequency ablation: a prospective comparison with nonsubcapsular liver tumors for safety and effectiveness. Radiology. 2008;248(2):670–9.
4. Song I, Rhim H, Lim HK, Kim YS, Choi D. Percutaneous radiofrequency ablation of hepatocellular carcinoma abutting the diaphragm and gastrointestinal tracts with the use of artificial ascites: safety and technical efficacy in 143 patients. Eur Radiol. 2009;19(11):2630–40.
5. Kang TW, Lim HK, Lee MW, Kim YS, Choi D, Rhim H. First-line radiofrequency ablation with or without artificial ascites for hepatocellular carcinomas in a subcapsular location: local control rate and risk of peritoneal seeding at long-term follow-up. Clin Radiol. 2013;68(12):e641–51.
6. Crucitti A, Danza FM, Antinori A, Vincenzo A, Pirulli PG, Bock E, Magistrelli P. Radiofrequency thermal ablation (RFA) of liver tumors: percutaneous and open surgical approaches. J Exp Clin Cancer Res. 2003;22(4 Suppl):191–5.
7. Santambrogio R, Podda M, Zuin M, Bertolini E, Bruno S, Cornalba GP, Costa M, Montorsi M. Safety and efficacy of laparoscopic radiofrequency ablation of hepatocellular carcinoma in patients with liver cirrhosis. Surg Endosc. 2003;17(11):1826–32.
8. Berber E, Siperstein AE. Perioperative outcome after laparoscopic radiofrequency ablation of liver tumors: an analysis of 521 cases. Surg Endosc. 2007;21(4):613–8.
9. Santambrogio R, Costa M, Barabino M, Opocher E. Laparoscopic radiofrequency of hepatocellular carcinoma using ultrasound-guided selective intrahepatic vascular occlusion. Surg Endosc. 2008;22(9):2051–5.
10. Birsen O, Aliyev S, Aksoy E, Taskin HE, Akyuz M, Karabulut K, Siperstein A, Berber E. A critical analysis of postoperative morbidity and mortality after laparoscopic radiofrequency ablation of liver tumors. Ann Surg Oncol. 2014;21(6):1834–40.
11. Schullian P, Weiss H, Klaus A, Widmann G, Kranewitter C, Mittermair C, Margreiter R, Bale R. Laparoscopic liver packing to protect surrounding organs during thermal ablation. Minim Invasive Ther Allied Technol. 2014;23(5):294–301.
12. Topal B, Hompes D, Aerts R, Fieuws S, Thijs M, Penninckx F. Morbidity and mortality of laparoscopic vs. open radiofrequency ablation for hepatic malignancies. Eur J Surg Oncol. 2007;33(5):603–7.
13. Tanaka S, Shimada M, Shirabe K, Taketomi A, Maehara S, Tsujita E, Ito S, Kitagawa D, Maehara Y. Surgical radiofrequency ablation for treatment of hepatocellular carcinoma: an endoscopic or open approach. Hepatogastroenterology. 2009;56(93):1169–73.
14. Sakoda M, Ueno S, Iino S, Minami K, Ando K, Kawasaki Y, Kurahara H, Mataki Y, Maemura K, Shinchi H, Natsugoe S. Endoscopic versus open radiofrequency ablation for treatment of small hepatocellular carcinoma. World J Surg. 2013;37(3):597–601.
15. Montorsi M, Santambrogio R, Bianchi P, Opocher E, Zuin M, Bertolini E, Bruno S, Podda M. Radiofrequency interstitial thermal ablation of hepatocellular carcinoma in liver cirrhosis. Role of the laparoscopic approach. Surg Endosc. 2001;15(2):141–5.
16. Hildebrand P, Kleemann M, Roblick U, Mirow L, Birth M, Bruch HP. Laparoscopic radiofrequency ablation of unresectable hepatic malignancies: indication, limitation and results. Hepatogastroenterology. 2007;54(79):2069–72.
17. Casaccia M, Andorno E, Nardi I, Santori G, Troilo B, Barabino G, Di Domenico S, Panaro F, Valente U. Laparoscopic staging and radiofrequency of hepatocellular carcinoma in liver cirrhosis. A "bridge" treatment to liver transplantation. Hepatogastroenterology. 2009;56(91–92):793–7.
18. Lee SD, Han HS, Cho JY, Yoon YS, Hwang DW, Jung K, Yoon CJ, Kwon Y, Kim JH. Safety and efficacy of laparoscopic radiofrequency ablation for hepatic malignancies. J Korean Surg Soc. 2012;83(1):36–42. Lap USG.
19. Jiang K, Zhang W, Su M, Liu Y, Zhao X, Wang J, Yao M, Ogbonna J, Dong J, Huang Z. Laparoscopic radiofrequency ablation of solitary small hepatocellular carcinoma in the caudate lobe. Eur J Surg Oncol. 2013;39(11):1236–42.
20. Machi J, Uchida S, Sumida K, Limm WM, Hundahl SA, Oishi AJ, Furumoto NL, Oishi RH. Ultrasound-guided radiofrequency thermal ablation of liver tumors: percutaneous, laparoscopic, and open surgical approaches. J Gastrointest Surg. 2001;5(5):477–89.
21. Santambrogio R, Opocher E, Costa M, Cappellani A, Montorsi M. Survival and intra-hepatic recurrences after laparoscopic radiofrequency of hepatocellular carcinoma in patients with liver cirrhosis. J Surg Oncol. 2005;89(4):218–25.
22. Salama IA, Korayem E, ElAbd O, El-Refaie A. Laparoscopic ultrasound with radiofrequency ablation of hepatic tumors in cirrhotic patients. J Laparoendosc Adv Surg Tech A. 2010;20(1):39–46.
23. Wong J, Lee KF, Yu SC, Lee PS, Cheung YS, Chong CN, Ip PC, Lai PB. Percutaneous radiofrequency ablation versus surgical radiofrequency ablation for malignant liver tumours: the long-term results. HPB (Oxford). 2013;15(8):595–601.

24. Herbold T, Wahba R, Bangard C, Demir M, Drebber U, Stippel DL. The laparoscopic approach for radiofrequency ablation of hepatocellular carcinoma--indication, technique and results. Langenbecks Arch Surg. 2013;398(1):47–53.

25. Karabulut K, Aucejo F, Akyildiz HY, Siperstein A, Berber E. Resection and radiofrequency ablation in the treatment of hepatocellular carcinoma: a single-center experience. Surg Endosc. 2012;26(4):990–7.

26. Santambrogio R, Opocher E, Zuin M, Selmi C, Bertolini E, Costa M, Conti M, Montorsi M. Surgical resection versus laparoscopic radiofrequency ablation in patients with hepatocellular carcinoma and Child-Pugh class a liver cirrhosis. Ann Surg Oncol. 2009;16(12):3289–98.

27. Lai EC, Tang CN. Radiofrequency ablation versus hepatic resection for hepatocellular carcinoma within the Milan criteria--a comparative study. Int J Surg. 2013;11(1):77–80.

28. Tohme S, Geller DA, Cardinal JS, Chen HW, Packiam V, Reddy S, Steel J, Marsh JW, Tsung A. Radiofrequency ablation compared to resection in early-stage hepatocellular carcinoma. HPB (Oxford). 2013;15(3):210–7.

# Peri-RFA Care and Management of Complications

**7**

Wan Yee Lau, Eric C.H. Lai, and Stephanie H.Y. Lau

## 7.1 Introduction

Radiofrequency ablation (RFA) to treat primary and secondary hepatic malignancies have gained widespread acceptance over the past 10 years. RFA of hepatic tumors can now be performed with low morbidity and mortality rates. Clinicians performing RFA must recognize early and late complications of RFA so as to intervene with appropriate treatment early.

The purpose of this chapter is to introduce the peri-RFA care. We also describe the complications of RFA, present tips and tricks to avoid or limit them, and introduce ways to appropriately manage them.

W.Y. Lau, MD, DSc, FACS, FRCS, FRACS(Hon) (✉)
Chinese Academy of Sciences, Faculty of Medicine,
The Chinese University of Hong Kong,
Shatin, New Territories, Hong Kong SAR, China
e-mail: josephlau@surgery.cuhk.edu.hk

E.C.H. Lai, MBChB(CUHK), MRCS(Ed), FRACS
Department of Surgery, Pamela Youde Nethersole
Eastern Hospital, Hong Kong SAR, China

S.H.Y. Lau, MBChB(CUHK), MRCS(Ed), FRCS(Ed)
Department of Surgery, Queen Elizabeth Hospital,
Hong Kong SAR, China

## 7.2 Peri-RFA Care

### 7.2.1 Pre-RFA Care

Before RFA, patients should routinely receive blood tests which include complete blood cell count, clotting profile, renal function test, hepatic function test, and tumor markers. For patients who have significant derangements in clotting profile or platelet count, fresh frozen plasma and platelets should be given before and/or during the procedure. Care should be taken to see whether patients are taking any anticoagulant. Warfarin should be converted to heparin, and all antiplatelet agents should be stopped at least a week before the procedure. In addition, a chest radiograph and abdominal computed tomography (CT) and/or magnetic resonance imaging (MRI) scan should be performed and reviewed. In patients with significant portal hypertension, upper gastrointestinal endoscopy is needed to assess, and to treat as appropriate, any esophageal and gastric varices. Patient education is an important part of the preparation. A thorough discussion and agreement on the treatment goals with the patients and their families should be done prior to the treatment.

The pre-RFA instructions will depend on whether RFA is performed under deep sedation or general anesthesia. Small quantities of water may be allowed up to 2 h prior to the procedure

© Springer Science+Business Media Dordrecht 2016
M. Chen et al. (eds.), *Radiofrequency Ablation for Small Hepatocellular Carcinoma*,
DOI 10.1007/978-94-017-7258-7_7

but nothing by mouth until after the patient wakes up from sedation or anesthesia. However, sedation and anesthesia guidelines may have local practice differences, and nothing by mouth for 6 h is practiced in some centers. Many clinicians routinely administer prophylactic antibiotics prior to RFA, although this is by no means universal and there is little strong evidence to support the practice.

For patients who are hepatitis B virus (HBV) surface antigen positive, reactivation of HBV happens quite commonly after systemic chemotherapy, transarterial chemoembolization (TACE), or hepatic resection for HBV-related hepatocellular carcinoma (HCC). However, the incidence of HBV reactivation and its significance on long-term survival after RFA in patients with HBV-related HCC are still unclear. There were only limited studies in this area. For patients with active HBV disease (such as elevated alanine aminotransferase (ALT) levels, positive HBeAg antigen, preoperative high HBV-DNA level), a medical hepatologist's assessment is necessary. In the retrospective study of Dan et al., 218 consecutive patients with HBV-related small HCC treated with RFA ($n = 125$) or hepatic resection ($n = 93$) from August 2006 to August 2011 were retrospectively studied. HBV reactivation developed in 20 (9.2 %) patients after treatment [1]. The incidence of HBV reactivation was significantly lower in the RFA group (5.6 %) than in the hepatic resection group (14.0 %). In the retrospective study of Xia et al., high levels of serum hyaluronic acid and HBV viral loads were the main prognostic factors of local recurrence after complete RFA for HBV-related small HCC [2]. The cumulative 1-, 3-, and 5-year disease-free survival rates were 86.8 %, 41.2 %, and 22.8 % in the high viral load group and 96.4 %, 65.8 %, and 36.7 % in the low viral load group, respectively. The difference between the two groups was significant. Based on the limited available evidences, it is still controversial to give routine prophylactic antiviral treatment for all HBV carriers before RFA. However, for those patients with a high preoperative HBV-DNA level, antiviral treatment is recommended.

### 7.2.2 RFA Procedure

RFA can be performed percutaneously, laparoscopically, or with open surgery. It involves placement of a thin needle electrode into the target tumor under ultrasound, CT, and/or MRI guidance. Grounding pads are placed on the patient and connected to a generator to create a complete electrical circuit. The needle electrode delivers alternating electrical current from the generator into the tumor and then to the dispersive electrodes (grounding pads). This causes local ionic agitation and subsequent frictional heat. Temperatures in excess of 50–60 °C cause irreversible thermal damage to the cells, termed coagulation necrosis. The by-products of the necrotic tissues are reabsorbed by the body, excreted via the kidneys, and replaced by scar tissues.

### 7.2.3 Post-RFA Care

Post-procedural instructions should include monitoring for vital signs, including temperature, oral intake and urine output, and skin integrity. Post-procedural resumption of diet depends on the usual anesthesia or sedation guidelines. Continued hydration is important to excrete the by-products of ablation via the kidney and limits renal toxicity or acute tubular necrosis from contrast or post-ablation syndrome. Pain medication should be given on demand by the patient. RFA at the dome of the liver near the diaphragm or near the liver capsule usually causes more pain, which can be at the treatment site or radiate to the right shoulder. Ablation size and proximity to the liver capsule have been related to the frequency and intensity of post-ablation pain. It is usually not severe and resolves in a few days. In addition, RFA at the dome of the liver has been associated with pleural effusion and requires close monitoring of the patient's respiratory status in the days and weeks following RFA. Patients may resume their normal levels of activity as tolerated, usually 24 h after RFA. There was no evidence to support the routine or selective use of post-RFA prophylactic antibiotics. However, antibiotic prophylaxis and possibly extended antibiotic coverage should be considered in high-risk patients with immunological impairment, ascites, history of bilioenteric anastomosis, or large ablative area.

Contrast CT scan is arranged 1 month after completion of the RFA therapy. If there is no evidence of residual tumor, CT scan is performed every 3 months to detect any residual or recurrence in the ablated tumor and to monitor for the development of new hepatic or extrahepatic disease. The image monitoring interval may be lengthened if there is no evidence of recurrence after the first 2 years of RFA.

## 7.3    Complications

The safety issue of RFA was established by a series of retrospective studies involving heterogeneous groups of patients with primary and secondary liver malignancies. In general, RFA is a safe procedure with very low rates of death and major complications. The reported mortality rate and major complication rate range from 0 % to 1.4 % and from 2.4 % to 12.7 %, respectively [3–11]. Complications resulting from RFA can be divided into two broad categories: complications secondary to RFA electrode placement and those secondary to thermal injury or tissue necrosis. The former category includes infection, bleeding, tumor seeding, and pneumothorax. The latter category includes post-ablation syndrome, thermal damage to adjacent organs, and grounding pad burns. Some complications occur more frequently with percutaneous RFA than with surgical RFA (e.g., gastrointestinal perforation, cholecystitis, pleural effusions, skin burns, tumor seeding).

### 7.3.1    Post-ablation Syndrome

The post-ablation syndrome is characterized as a self-limited flu-like illness with low-grade fever, malaise, nausea, and/or vomiting. The etiology of post-ablation syndrome has not been definitively determined. It is thought to be mediated by an inflammatory response to

necrotic tissues that results from ablation. The occurrence is observed in approximately one-third of patients [12, 13].

### 7.3.2    Grounding Pad Burns

Skin burns were frequently reported in the early series but have become rare since the introduction of modern systems using grounding plates with a much larger surface. Proper placement of grounding pads is very important or get skin burned (Fig. 7.1).

### 7.3.3    Intraperitoneal Bleeding

Bleeding complications are more likely to happen in patients with HCC due to their underlying liver diseases. The bleeding can present in the form of subcapsular hematoma, abdominal wall hematoma, intrahepatic parenchymal hematoma, or even hemoperitoneum [14–16]. It is important to select a needle electrode path that traverses sufficient normal liver parenchyma to avoid hepatic vessels while positioning the needle electrode and to perform cauterization of the needle electrode track after ablation. Increasing abdominal pain following the procedure is generally the most common symptom. Repeat hemoglobin level, ultrasound, or CT scan confirms the diagnosis. Although most minor bleeding after RFA stops spontane-

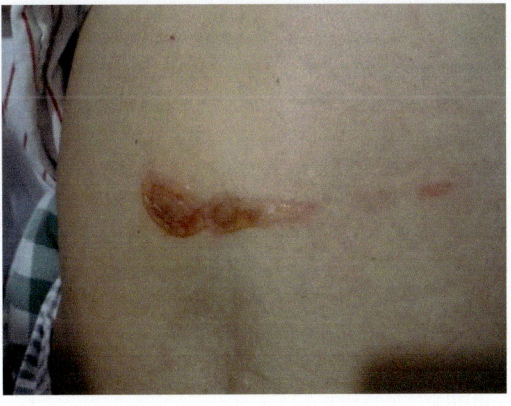

**Fig. 7.1**   Grounding pad burns after RFA

ously, close clinical evaluation of a patient's vital signs and laboratory tests immediately after ablation are essential for early detection and proper management of this potentially life-threatening complication (e.g., fluid resuscitation, blood transfusion, correction of coagulopathy). Venous bleeding sometimes stops by itself. Uncontrolled arterial bleeding or pseudoaneurysm formation needs to have trans-femoral hepatic arterial branch embolization to control the bleeding. If bleeding is not controlled by non-surgical means, surgical intervention is needed.

### 7.3.4 Hepatic Failure

Liver failure is also a potentially fatal complication, especially in patients with cirrhosis whose liver function is already impaired. Similar to post-hepatectomy patients, there are multiple risk factors for the development of this severe complication, such as insufficient liver functional remnant, vascular thrombosis, major biliary injury, liver abscess, or sepsis due to intestinal perforation.

### 7.3.5 Intrahepatic Abscess

Secondary bacterial contamination of the ablated hepatic parenchyma may lead to abscess formation. The presence of biliary-enteric communication at the time of the procedure has been noted to significantly increase the risk of abscess formation [17]. It can be difficult to differentiate fever as a component of the post-ablation syndrome from that secondary to an intrahepatic abscess. This difficulty may delay the diagnosis. The possibility of abscess formation should be considered if the fever pattern is high and swinging or lasts longer than 1 week because fever in the post-ablation syndrome usually is low grade and lasts less than 1 week. Most abscesses can be successfully managed by simple aspiration or percutaneous catheter drainage coupled with adequate antibiotics coverage.

### 7.3.6 Bile Duct Injury

Biliary tract damage includes biliary stricture; bilomas; and, rarely, bilio-peritoneum and bilio-pleural fistula. The proximity of liver tumor to the right or left hepatic ducts, or sectoral bile ducts, increases the risk of biliary stricture or biliary fistula due to thermal induced necrosis and/or direct ductal puncture. Most of these changes have no clinical significance with the patient being asymptomatic, and major complications requiring additional treatment are rare. While biliary stricture has no clinical significance when it is located peripherally, it is sometimes troublesome when located centrally in the major bile ducts. Bile duct cooling using an endoscopic nasobiliary drainage (ENBD) tube during RFA for HCC close to major bile ducts has been reported to be safe and feasible [18–20]. This technique increases the indications of RFA in difficult cases. Another complication is hemobilia, which is caused by the simultaneous puncture of the biliary tract and a vessel. The most common symptoms are abdominal pain, hematemesis, and melena.

RFA of tumors adjacent to the gallbladder is often accompanied by a high risk of gallbladder perforation or acute cholecystitis due to thermal injury. Therefore, when treating tumors adjacent to the gallbladder, an open or laparoscopic technique provides the chance to perform prophylactic cholecystectomy, thus decreasing the risk.

### 7.3.7 Vascular Thrombosis

Portal vein thrombosis, hepatic vein thrombosis, hepatic artery damage, and pseudoaneurysm represent this group of complications. Heat-related vascular thrombosis is only observed in vessels smaller than 3 mm and has no symptomatic consequences. Larger caliber vessels are protected by the continuous cooling effect of blood flow. Most of these thromboses are asymptomatic even in large vessels, and no further therapy is required. In general, thrombi within portal and hepatic veins require no specific therapy if liver function is unaffected. They are caused by heat damage to the endothelial cells of the portal or hepatic vein, leading to platelet aggregation and subsequent thrombosis.

## 7.3.8 Gastrointestinal Tract Injury

Liver tumors are sometimes adjacent to the stomach, ascending colon, and duodenum. When a liver tumor is close to the gastrointestinal tract, the gastrointestinal tract should be displaced away from the tumor to avoid thermal injury from RFA. Tumors that lie adjacent to the gastrointestinal tract may be protected by changing the patient's body position, interposition of induced ascites, or aspirating gas inside the bowel [21]. If safe displacement of the gastrointestinal tract is not feasible, laparoscopic or open approach of RFA should be considered. Early diagnosis and adequate treatment of thermal injury to the gastrointestinal tract are essential since it may lead to death.

## 7.3.9 Thoracic Complications

Pneumothorax, hemothorax, pleural effusions, and pneumonia are in this group of complications. For liver tumors which are located near the hepatic dome, the diaphragm is particularly exposed to the risk of thermal injury; the consequences are generally limited to a reactive pleural effusion or to a more intense and prolonged pain syndrome. Delayed diaphragmatic hernia can occur as a result of this thermal injury, and these patients can be asymptomatic or present with acute bowel strangulation [22, 23].

Several authors have also described hemothorax as a complication of percutaneous RFA. It is less frequent than intra-abdominal bleeding. It usually occurs when an intercostal approach is used to carry out RFA for patients with tumors in the right liver, with injuries to intercostal arteries. Diaphragmatic muscle hemorrhage has also been reported during trans-diaphragmatic approach of RFA using artificial hydrothorax for subdiaphragmatic liver malignancies [24]. Chest pain and dyspnea are the most common symptoms. Ultrasound, CT scan, and chest X-ray confirm the diagnosis.

## 7.3.10 Tumor Seeding

Tumor seeding in the needle tract has been reported with an incidence varying from 0.6 % to 4 % [25–30]. Viable tumor cells adherent to a biopsy needle or a RFA needle electrode which drop off during needle extraction, tumor cells which are carried into the needle tract during bleeding, or tumor cells which are forced into the needle tract by intratumoral hyperpressure created by the RFA process are the mechanisms that explain tumor seeding (Fig. 7.2). Decreasing the number of punctures and transversing a large amount of liver parenchyma before entering the tumor may prevent this complication. Indirect punctures through an area of healthy liver parenchyma and coagulation of the needle tract are recommended to reduce the risk of bleeding and tumor implantation, especially for subcapsular lesions. Other risks factors reported are poor tumor differentiation, subcapsular location (where heating of the needle tract is not possible), previous biopsy before RFA, and multiple needle insertions. Therefore, an optimal and meticulous first attempt in the needle electrode positioning is desirable.

### Conclusion

Careful patient selection, choice of the most appropriate imaging modality and approach, followed by early detection and appropriate management should a complication occur help to minimize the incidence of complication and the degree of morbidity of RFA. Clinicians utilizing RFA to treat liver tumors must be aware that treatment-related complications can develop even months after the treatment.

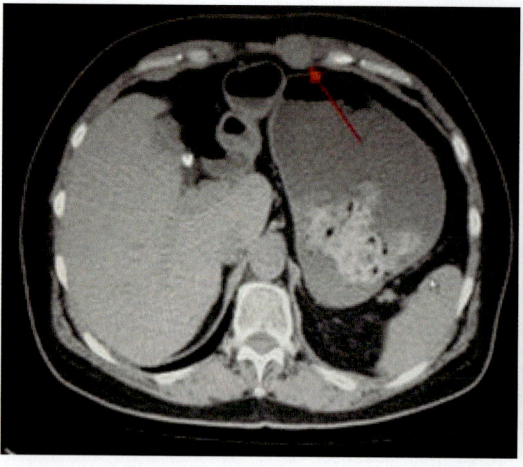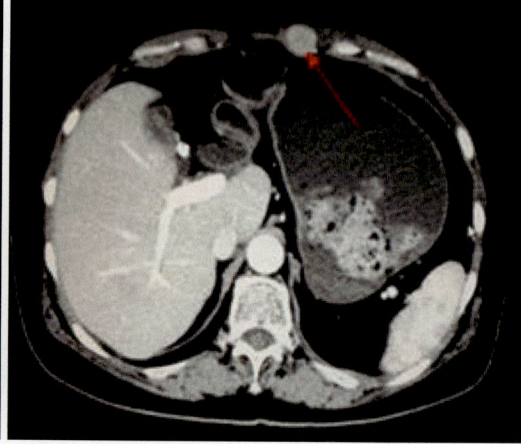

**Fig. 7.2** Tumor (*arrows*) seeding to abdomen wall after RFA

# References

1. Dan JQ, Zhang YJ, Huang JT, Chen MS, Gao HJ, Peng ZW, Xu L, Lau WY. Hepatitis B virus reactivation after radiofrequency ablation or hepatic resection for HBV-related small hepatocellular carcinoma: a retrospective study. Eur J Surg Oncol. 2013;39(8):865–72.

2. Xia F, Lai EC, Lau WY, Ma K, Li X, Bie P, Qian C. High serum hyaluronic acid and HBV viral load are main prognostic factors of local recurrence after complete radiofrequency ablation of hepatitis B-related small hepatocellular carcinoma. Ann Surg Oncol. 2012;19(4):1284–91.

3. Curley SA, Izzo F, Ellis LM, Nicolas Vauthey J, Vallone P. Radiofrequency ablation of hepatocellular cancer in 110 patients with cirrhosis. Ann Surg. 2000;232(3):381–91.

4. Mulier S, Mulier P, Ni Y, Miao Y, Dupas B, Marchal G, De Wever I, Michel L. Complications of radiofrequency coagulation of liver tumours. Br J Surg. 2002;89(10):1206–22.

5. Rhim H, Yoon KH, Lee JM, Cho Y, Cho JS, Kim SH, Lee WJ, Lim HK, Nam GJ, Han SS, Kim YH, Park CM, Kim PN, Byun JY. Major complications after radio-frequency thermal ablation of hepatic tumors: spectrum of imaging findings. Radiographics. 2003;23(1):123–34.

6. Chen MH, Yan K, Yang W, Gao W, Dai Y, Wang YB, Zhang H, Huo L, Xing BC, Huang XF. Efficacy of radiofrequency ablation of 343 patients with hepatic tumor and the relevant complications. Beijing Da Xue Xue Bao. 2005;37(3):292–6.

7. Poggi G, Riccardi A, Quaretti P, Teragni C, Delmonte A, Amatu A, Saini G, Mazzucco M, Bernardo A, Palumbo R, Canto A, Bernieri S, Bernardo G. Complications of percutaneous radiofrequency

thermal ablation of primary and secondary lesions of the liver. Anticancer Res. 2007;27(4C):2911–6.

8. Kasugai H, Osaki Y, Oka H, Kudo M, Seki T, Osaka Liver Cancer Study Group. Severe complications of radiofrequency ablation therapy for hepatocellular carcinoma: an analysis of 3,891 ablations in 2,614 patients. Oncology. 2007;72 Suppl 1:72–5.

9. Koda M, Murawaki Y, Hirooka Y, Kitamoto M, Ono M, Sakaeda H, Joko K, Sato S, Tamaki K, Yamasaki T, Shibata H, Shimoe T, Matsuda T, Toshikuni N, Fujioka S, Ohmoto K, Nakamura S, Kariyama K, Aikata H, Kobayashi Y, Tsutsui A. Complications of radiofrequency ablation for hepatocellular carcinoma in a multicenter study: an analysis of 16346 treated nodules in 13283 patients. Hepatol Res. 2012;42(11):1058–64.

10. Takaki H, Yamakado K, Nakatsuka A, Yamada T, Shiraki K, Takei Y, Takeda K. Frequency of and risk factors for complications after liver radiofrequency ablation under CT fluoroscopic guidance in 1500 sessions: single-center experience. AJR Am J Roentgenol. 2013;200(3):658–64.

11. de Baère T, Risse O, Kuoch V, Dromain C, Sengel C, Smayra T, Gamal El Din M, Letoublon C, Elias D. Adverse events during radiofrequency treatment of 582 hepatic tumors. AJR Am J Roentgenol. 2003;181(3):695–700.

12. Dodd 3rd GD, Napier D, Schoolfield JD, Hubbard L. Percutaneous radiofrequency ablation of hepatic tumors: postablation syndrome. AJR Am J Roentgenol. 2005;185:51–7.

13. Carrafiello G, Laganà D, Ianniello A, Dionigi G, Novario R, Recaldini C, Mangini M, Cuffari S, Fugazzola C. Post-radiofrequency ablation syndrome after percutaneous radiofrequency of abdominal tumours: one centre experience and review of published works. Australas Radiol. 2007;51(6):550–4.

14. Goto E, Tateishi R, Shiina S, Masuzaki R, Enooku K, Sato T, Ohki T, Kondo Y, Goto T, Yoshida H, Omata

M. Hemorrhagic complications of percutaneous radiofrequency ablation for liver tumors. J Clin Gastroenterol. 2010;44(5):374–80.

15. Chen MH, Dai Y, Yan K, Yang W, Gao W, Wu W, Liao SR, Hao CY. Intraperitoneal hemorrhage during and after percutaneous radiofrequency ablation of hepatic tumors: reasons and management. Chin Med J (Engl). 2005;118(20):1682–7.

16. Minami Y, Hayaishi S, Kudo M. Radiofrequency ablation for hepatic malignancies: is needle tract cauterization necessary for preventing iatrogenic bleeding? Dig Dis. 2013;31(5–6):480–4.

17. Birsen O, Aliyev S, Aksoy E, Taskin HE, Akyuz M, Karabulut K, Siperstein A, Berber E. A critical analysis of postoperative morbidity and mortality after laparoscopic radiofrequency ablation of liver tumors. Ann Surg Oncol. 2014;21(6):1834–40.

18. Ohnishi T, Yasuda I, Nishigaki Y, Hayashi H, Otsuji K, Mukai T, Enya M, Omar S, Soehendra N, Tomita E, Moriwaki H. Intraductal chilled saline perfusion to prevent bile duct injury during percutaneous radiofrequency ablation for hepatocellular carcinoma. J Gastroenterol Hepatol. 2008;23(8 Pt 2):e410–5.

19. Nakata Y, Haji S, Ishikawa H, Yasuda T, Nakai T, Takeyama Y, Shiozaki H. Two cases of hepatocellular carcinoma located adjacent to the Glisson's capsule treated by laparoscopic radiofrequency ablation with intraductal chilled saline perfusion through an endoscopic nasobiliary drainage tube. Surg Laparosc Endosc Percutan Tech. 2010;20(6):e189–92.

20. Kurihara N, Kato H, Hirao K, Mizuno O, Ishida E, Okada H, Yamamoto K. Prevention of biliary complication in radiofrequency ablation for hepatocellular carcinoma-Cooling effect by endoscopic nasobiliary drainage tube. Eur J Radiol. 2010;73:385–90.

21. Hirooka M, Kisaka Y, Uehara T, Ishida K, Kumagi T, Watanabe Y, Abe M, Matsuura B, Hiasa Y, Onji M. Efficacy of laparoscopic radiofrequency ablation for hepatocellular carcinoma compared to percutaneous radiofrequency ablation with artificial ascites. Dig Endosc. 2009;21(2):82–6.

22. Kim JS, Kim HS, Myung DS, Lee GH, Park KJ, Cho SB, Joo YE, Choi SK. A case of diaphragmatic hernia induced by radiofrequency ablation for hepatocellular carcinoma. Korean J Gastroenterol. 2013;62(3): 174–8.

23. Nakamura T, Masuda K, Thethi RS, Sako H, Yoh T, Nakao T, Yoshimura N. Successful surgical rescue of delayed onset diaphragmatic hernia following radiofrequency ablation for hepatocellular carcinoma. Ulus Travma Acil Cerrahi Derg. 2014;20(4):295–9.

24. Han Y, Yu L, Hao YZ, Yang M, Liu S, Deng YB, He LF, Cai JQ, Chen MH. Percutaneous radiofrequency ablation with artificial hydrothorax for liver cancer in the hepatic dome. Zhonghua Zhong Liu Za Zhi. 2012;34(11):846–9.

25. Llovet JM, Vilana R, Brú C, Bianchi L, Salmeron JM, Boix L, Ganau S, Sala M, Pagès M, Ayuso C, Solé M, Rodés J, Bruix J, Barcelona Clínic Liver Cancer (BCLC) Group. Increased risk of tumor seeding after percutaneous radiofrequency ablation for single hepatocellular carcinoma. Hepatology. 2001;33(5): 1124–9.

26. Jaskolka JD, Asch MR, Kachura JR, Ho CS, Ossip M, Wong F, Sherman M, Grant DR, Greig PD, Gallinger S. Needle tract seeding after radiofrequency ablation of hepatic tumors. J Vasc Interv Radiol. 2005;16(4):485–91.

27. Livraghi T, Lazzaroni S, Meloni F, Solbiati L. Risk of tumour seeding after percutaneous radiofrequency ablation for hepatocellular carcinoma. Br J Surg. 2005;92:856–8.

28. Perkins JD. Seeding risk following percutaneous approach to hepatocellular carcinoma. Liver Transpl. 2007;13(11):1603.

29. Imamura J, Tateishi R, Shiina S, Goto E, Sato T, Ohki T, Masuzaki R, Goto T, Yoshida H, Kanai F, Hamamura K, Obi S, Yoshida H, Omata M. Neoplastic seeding after radiofrequency ablation for hepatocellular carcinoma. Am J Gastroenterol. 2008;103:3057–62.

30. Latteri F, Sandonato L, Di Marco V, Parisi P, Cabibbo G, Lombardo G, Galia M, Midiri M, Latteri MA, Craxì A. Seeding after radiofrequency ablation of hepatocellular carcinoma in patients with cirrhosis: a prospective study. Dig Liver Dis. 2008;40(8):684–9.

# Combined Therapies of RFA

**8**

Zhenwei Peng and Minshan Chen

## 8.1 Introduction

RFA has been widely utilized in the treatment of small HCC (≤3 cm) with encouraging results. However, the limited volume of coagulative necrosis obtained with RFA systems and the occasionally irregular burn shape caused by the heat sink activity of the large vessels in the proximity of the ablated area have prevented the widespread use of RFA in the treatment of hepatic tumors. To obtain a large coagulation area, various techniques including transcatheter arterial chemoembolization (TACE), percutaneous ethanol injection (PEI), balloon occlusion of the hepatic artery and saline infusion during RFA, and so on have been used.

## 8.2 TACE Combined with RFA

Nowadays, RFA is generally recognized as an alternative treatment to partial hepatectomy for early HCC (solitary tumor ≤5.0 cm in diameter or fewer than 3 nodules ≤3.0 cm in diameter),

Z. Peng, MD, PhD
Department of Oncology, The First Affiliated Hospital of Sun Yat-sen University, Guangzhou, China

M. Chen, MD, PhD (✉)
Department of Hepatobiliary Surgery, Sun Yat-sen University Cancer Center, Guangzhou, China
e-mail: chminsh@mail.sysu.edu.cn

especially for patients with impaired liver function and when liver transplantation is not indicated, although some authors consider that RFA can be used as a first-line treatment for early HCC. However, the likelihood of complete ablation using RFA declines rapidly as tumor diameter increases [1]. The complete response rate after RFA for HCC 2.0 cm is over 90 %, but the local failure rate in individuals with HCC between 3.1 and 4.0 cm may be 24 % with patients treated with RFA, and the likelihood of complete ablation rapidly declines beyond 4 cm [2]. TACE can slow tumor progression and improves survival by combining the effect of targeted chemotherapy with ischemic necrosis by arterial embolization. Although TACE is most commonly classified as palliative rather than potentially curative, there is evidence that TACE prolongs survival in patients with well-compensated liver disease and intermediate-stage HCC. Because blood flow promotes heat loss and heat loss may reduce the effectiveness of RFA, a possible way to increase the ablation size of RFA thermal lesions would be to reduce or eliminate the heat loss that is mediated by tissue perfusion [3]. Blood flow to HCC lesions can be substantially reduced by the arterial embolization effect of TACE treatment. Moreover, TACE has a strong antitumor effect on HCC lesions. The synergy between TACE and RFA is well described [3]. Occlusion of hepatic arterial flow by embolization reduces the cooling effect of hepatic blood

© Springer Science+Business Media Dordrecht 2016
M. Chen et al. (eds.), *Radiofrequency Ablation for Small Hepatocellular Carcinoma*,
DOI 10.1007/978-94-017-7258-7_8

flow on thermal coagulation. Furthermore, iodized oil and gelatin sponge particles used in TACE fill the peripheral portal vein around the tumor by going through multiple arterioportal communications, thus reducing the portal venous flow [3]. As a consequence, RFA can enable the creation of larger thermal lesions by RFA (Figs. 8.1 and 8.2).

The effect of chemotherapeutic anticancer agents on cancer cells enhances the effect of hyperthermia [4]. TACE, being a regional treatment, can target undetected satellite lesions outside of the zone of RFA-induced necrosis. Moreover, disruption of intratumoral septa, which usually happens after TACE, facilitates heat distribution within the tumor, and intratumoral septa and fibrosis are considered to hamper heat diffusion within the tumor [4]. Sequential application of TACE and RFA is, therefore, increasingly being used in the treatment of HCC in patients with well-compensated liver disease.

Recently, TACE-RFA has been reported to be an effective and safe treatment for HCC [5–11] (Table 8.1).

The way of enhancing the efficacy of RFA by TACE is to decrease the blood flow of the tumor area to be ablated with subsequent decrease in heat loss by convection. Several studies have demonstrated the synergistic cytotoxic effects of TACE with RFA for the treatment of HCC, especially for medium-sized HCC (3–5 cm). The procedure for TACE-RFA is TACE first followed by RFA within 1 month. A recently published randomized controlled trial by Shibata et al. demonstrated a survival equality for combined TACE and RFA ($n=46$) compared with RFA alone ($n=43$) in patients with Child's A or B cirrhosis and resectable HCC with ≤3 nodules smaller than 3 cm [5]. In this study, after treatment, the 1-, 2-, 3-, and 4-year rates of local tumor progression, overall survival, local progression-free survival, and recurrence-free survival were as

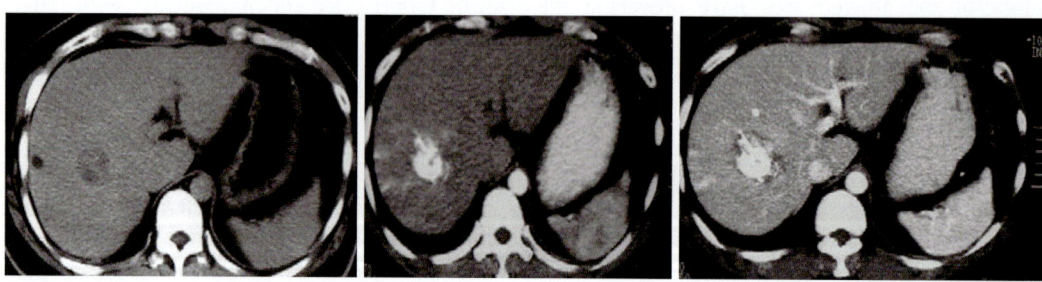

**Fig. 8.1** sHCC treated by TACE+RFA

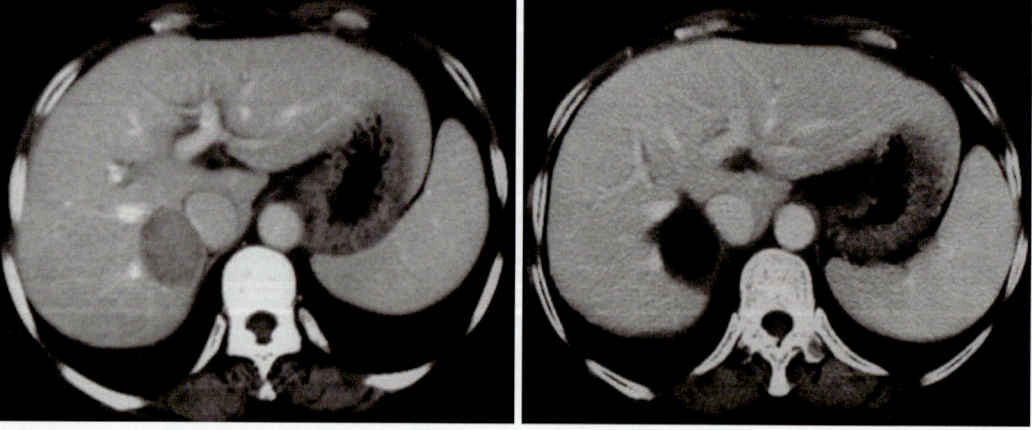

**Fig. 8.2** sHCC treated by PEI+RFA

**Table 8.1** Trials to compare TACE-RFA with RFA alone

| Ref. | Design | Treatment | No. of patients | Recurrence-free survival rate | | | Overall survival rate | | |
|------|--------|-----------|-----------------|-------------------------------|---|---|-----------------------|---|---|
| | | | | 1 year (%) | 3 years | 5 years | 1 year (%) | 3 years | 5 years |
| Shibata et al. [5] | RCT | TACE-RFA | 46 | 71.30 | 48.80 % | NA | 100.00 | 84.8 % | NA |
| | | RFA | 43 | 74.30 | 29.70 % | NA | 100.00 | 84.50 % | NA |
| Morimoto et al. [6] | RCT | TACE-RFA | 19 | 67.00 | NA | NA | 100.00 | 93.00 % | NA |
| | | RFA | 18 | 56.00 | 28.00 % | NA | 89.00 | 80.00 % | NA |
| Peng et al. [7] | RCT | TACE-RFA | 94 | 79.4 | 60.6 % | NA | 92.6 | 66.6 % | NA |
| | | RFA | 95 | 66.7 | 44.2 | NA | 85.3 | 59 % | NA |
| Yang et al. [8] | Cohort | TACE-RFA | 24 | 29.00 | NA | NA | 68.00 | NA | NA |
| | | RFA | 12 | 34.70 | NA | NA | 57.00 | NA | NA |
| Shen et al. [9] | Cohort | TACE-RFA | 18 | 63.90 | 50.00 % | NA | 87.50 | 73.30 % | NA |
| | | RFA | 16 | 30.00 | 18.70 % | NA | 52.20 | 20.40 % | NA |

*NA* not applicable

follows: local tumor progression rates were 14.4 %, 17.6 %, 17.6 %, and 17.6 %, respectively, in the combined treatment group and 11.4 %, 14.4 %, 14.4 %, and 14.4 %, respectively, in the RFA group ($P=0.797$). Overall survival rates were 100 %, 100 %, 84.8 %, and 72.7 %, respectively, in the combined treatment group and 100 %, 88.8 %, 84.5 %, and 74.0 %, respectively, in the RFA group ($P=0.515$). Local progression-free survival rates were 84.6 %, 81.1 %, 69.7 %, and 55.8 %, respectively, in the combined treatment group and 88.4 %, 74.1 %, 74.1 %, and 61.7 %, respectively, in the RFA group ($P=0.934$). Event-free survival rates were 71.3 %, 59.9 %, 48.8 %, and 36.6 %, respectively, in the combined treatment group and 74.3 %, 52.4 %, 29.7 %, and 29.7 %, respectively, in the RFA group ($P=0.365$). In light of this study, the authors considered that combined RFA plus TACE and RFA alone have equivalent effectiveness for the treatment of small (≤3 cm) HCCs, and they thought the combination treatment may not be necessary. In the study, both treatment groups had low rates of major complications (2.2–2.3 %), and it was stated that treatment of HCC by combined TACE and RFA was safe. Morimoto et al. reported the midterm outcomes of a randomized controlled trial comparing the efficacy of TACE combined with RFA with RFA alone for the treatment of intermediate-sized HCC [6]. In the study, the authors randomly assigned 37 patients with solitary HCCs (diameter 3.1–5.0 cm in the greatest dimension) to two groups: the TACE combined with RFA (TACE-RFA) group and the RFA group. The results showed that technical success was achieved after $1.4\pm0.5$ RFA sessions in the RFA group and after $1.1\pm0.2$ RFA sessions in the TACE-RFA group ($P=0.01$). The mean diameters of the longer and shorter axes of the RFA-induced ablated were $50\pm8.0$ and $41\pm7.1$ mm, respectively, in the RFA group and $58\pm13.2$ and $50\pm11.3$ mm, respectively, in the TACE-RFA group; the mean diameters of the shorter axes were significantly different ($P=0.012$). The rates of local tumor progression at the end of the third year in the RFA and TACE-RFA groups were 39 and 6 %, respectively ($P=0.012$). The 3-year survival rates of the patients in the RFA and TACE-RFA groups were 80 and 93 %, respectively ($P=0.369$). The authors reported that TACE prior to RFA expanded the short axis of the ablated area and resulted in a more spherical ablated area. They postulated that a spherical ablated area was more effective than a nonspherical ablated area in ensuring local tumor control because a spherical ablated area was more likely to completely cover the target tumor. TACE-RFA was also a safe treatment in this study. The result showed that there were no severe side effects during the procedures in the study; however, six patients (five patients of the RFA group and one patient of the TACE-RFA group) experienced grade 1–2 pain lasting several hours. Major complications were not observed in the patients of the two groups. Minor complications, including asymptomatic right pleural effusion, were noted within 3 days of the procedures in two patients of the RFA group and one patient of the TACE-RFA group (RFA group vs. TACE-RFA group, $P=0.515$). Recently, a randomized controlled trial published by Peng et al. demonstrated that the survival benefit for combined TACE and RFA ($n=94$) was comparable with RFA alone ($n=95$) in patients with Child's A or B cirrhosis and resectable HCC with ≤3 nodules smaller than 7.0 cm [7]. In this study, after treatment, the 1-, 3-, and 4-year overall survival rates for the TACE-RFA group and the RFA group were 92.6 %, 66.6 %, and 61.8 % and 85.3 %, 59 %, and 45.0 %, respectively. The corresponding recurrence-free survival rates were 79.4 %, 60.6 %, and 54.8 % and 66.7 %, 44.2 %, and 38.9 %, respectively. Patients in the TACE-RFA group had better overall survival and recurrence-free survival than the RFA group ($P=0.002$ and 0.009, respectively). After multivariate analysis, treatment allocation, tumor size, and tumor number were significant prognostic factors for overall survival, while treatment allocation and tumor number were significant prognostic factors for recurrence-free survival. There were no treatment-related deaths in this study. In light of this study, the role of combined TACE and RFA warrants careful consideration. The study provides evidence that altering the tumor microenvironment and supporting vasculature may help improve the efficacy of locoregional therapy in HCC.

Recently, some authors have used meta-analysis to verify the role of TACE combined with RFA in the treatment of HCC. In Yan's studies, four randomized control trials were included into the meta-analysis [10]. Meta-analyses showed that the combination of RFA and TACE was associated with higher survival rates (1-year OR = 2.14, 95 % CI 1.57–2.91, $P=0.001$; 3-year OR = 1.98, 95 % CI 1.28–3.07, $P=0.001$; 5-year OR = 2.70, 95 % CI 1.42–.14, $P=0.003$). They postulate that the combination of TACE with RFA can improve the overall survival rate and provide better prognosis for patients with HCC, but more randomized controlled trials using large sample size are needed to provide sufficient evidence. In another meta-analysis study,

Wang et al. reported that there was no survival benefit from TACE combined with RFA in treating small HCC (≤3 cm) patients as compared with that of RFA alone [11]. The advantages of TACE-RFA may be as follows: TACE can block the hepatic arterial flow and contribute to the decrease in heat sink effects and the increase in the necrotic area induced by RFA, and the effect of anticancer agents on cancer cells may be enhanced by the hyperthermia. However, these advantages do not seem to have any indication according to Wang et al. meta-analysis for small HCC [11]. The reason for this may be that RFA has already achieved complete necrosis in >90 % in treating small HCC nodules, suggesting that adding TACE to RFA seems to be redundant in producing an assessed outcome. Schwartz and Weintraub considered that the clearest role for the combination of TACE and RFA is to increase the likelihood of complete destruction of HCC nodules that are in the range of 3–5 cm [12]. They also say that patients selected for combined TACE and RFA should have well-compensated cirrhosis and the rationale for using combined therapy is strongest for patients with uninodular HCC. Therefore, the role of TACE combined with RFA in the treatment of HCC needs further study.

TACE combined with RFA can also improve the efficacy of recurrent HCC after curative treatment [8, 13]. Yang et al. conducted a study to assess the efficacy and safety of RFA combined with TACE in recurrent HCC after hepatectomy and to compare its outcome with a single modality in recent year [8]. In this study, 103 patients with recurrent HCCs after hepatectomy who were excluded from repeat hepatectomy were allocated to three groups according to treatment modality. RFA was used as the sole first-line anticancer treatment in 37 patients (RFA group); TACE was used as the sole first-line anticancer treatment in 35 patients (TACE group). RFA followed by TACE was performed in 31 patients (combination group). There was no significant difference in clinical material between the three groups. The treatment success rate of the combination group was significantly higher than that of the TACE group (93.5 % vs. 68.6 %, $P=0.011$). The intrahepatic recurrence rate of the combination group was significantly lower than that of the TACE group (20.7 % vs. 57.1 %, $P=0.002$) and the RFA group (20.7 % vs. 43.2 %, $P=0.036$). The overall 1-, 3-, and 5-year survival rates were 73.9 %, 51.1 %, and 28.0 %, respectively, in the RFA group; 65.8 %, 38.9 %, and 19.5 %, respectively, in the TACE group; and 88.5 %, 64.6 %, and 44.3 %, respectively, in the combination group. There was a significant difference in survival between the combination group and the TACE group ($P=0.028$). Only one case of hemothorax was found in the combination group and recovered after percutaneous drainage. They thought that RFA combined with TACE was more effective in treating recurrent HCC after hepatectomy compared to single RFA or TACE treatment. This combination therapy can thus be a valuable choice of treatment for recurrent HCC. This study was limited by a possible selection bias resulting from the comparison of these nonrandomized groups and retrospective profile. Second, the number of TACE courses in each case was not strictly defined, because of repetitions planned on the basis of tumor response and patient tolerance. The best way to confirm this study's result is to conduct randomized control trials. Peng et al. conducted a randomized study and try to figure out whether TACE combined sequentially with RFA is more effective than RFA alone for the treatment of HCC recurrence after curative treatment [13]. From January 2002 to December 2006, 139 patients with recurrent HCC $\leq 5$ cm were randomized to receive either sequential TACE-RFA ($n=69$) or RFA alone ($n=70$). During follow-up, 32 patients in sequential treatment group and 35 patients in RFA group died. There was no significant difference between sequential treatment group and RFA group in terms of local tumor progression (1/69 vs. 2/70, $P=0.576$). This prospective study showed that overall survival and recurrence-free survival for sequential TACE-RFA were significantly better than that for RFA alone ($P=0.037$, $P=0.005$, respectively). On subgroup analyses, the overall survival and recurrence-free survival for sequential TACE-RFA group were better than that for RFA group for patients with intervals of tumor recurrence from the initial treatment being

$\leq 1$ year ($P=0.004$, $P=0.020$, respectively) for tumors 3.1–5.0 cm in diameter ($P=0.002$, $P<0.001$, respectively). A logistic regression analysis showed that the interval of tumor recurrence from the initial treatment and treatment allocation were significant prognostic factors for overall survival, while the interval of tumor recurrence from the initial treatment, treatment allocation, and tumor size were significant prognostic factors for recurrence-free survival. According to this study, sequential TACE-RFA treatment has better efficacy than RFA for recurrent HCC $\leq 5$ cm. For patients with 3–5 cm tumors or patients with interval of tumor recurrence from the initial treatment of $\leq 1$ year, sequential TACE-RFA treatment should be recommended.

## 8.3 Combined with Percutaneous Ethanol Injection (PEI)

PEI had been utilized in the treatment of HCC for a long time. It usually requires to be repeated several times and with the disadvantages of long treatment cycle, high local recurrence rate, etc. RFA-PEI is also an effective combined treatment for HCC. Studies have demonstrated that RFA-PEI is able to achieve a larger ablative zone than RFA, which will lead to lower local recurrence rate and better survivals [14] (Figs. 8.2 and 8.3).

The procedure for RFA-PEI is RFA needle and PEI needle are inserted into the tumor at the same time, absolute alcohol is injected first, and then RFA is performed minutes after PEI. During RFA combined with PEI therapy (PEI followed by RFA), the injected ethanol embolizes vessels $\leq 5$ mm, so that blood infusion is reduced. Meanwhile, the ethanol can disperse to area which RFA failed to reach, such as perivascular tumors. In this way, the ablative effect is enhanced. In Zhang et al. RCT, 133 patients were randomly assigned to receive RFA-PEI ($n=66$) or RFA alone ($n=67$) [14]. The 5-year overall survival rates for the RFA-PEI group and the RFA alone group were 49.3 % and 35.9 %, respectively. The RFA-PEI offered significant

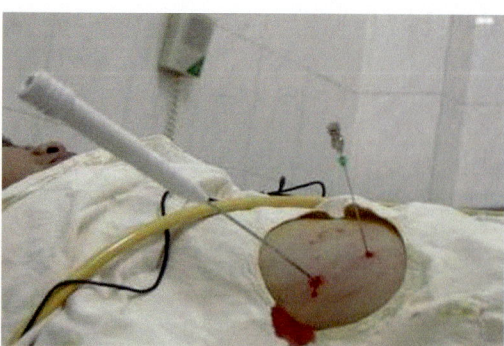

**Fig. 8.3** Procedure for PEI+RFA

survival advantage over RFA alone for patients with tumors of 3.1–5.0 cm in diameter but not for those with tumors equal or less than 3.0 cm in diameter, or for those with tumors 5.1–7.0 cm in diameter. Moreover, some reports have suggested that RFA combined with injection of cytotoxic drugs will improve the efficacy although this remains to be proved.

PEI can be useful when tumors are in close vicinity (<1 cm) to vital structures, including biliary ducts, stomach, intestinal loops, and kidney, and whose location makes them difficult to treat with thermal ablative techniques. In addition, PEI is useful for lesions that remain undetected by ultrasound, such as masses in the hepatic dome or small nodules, or when the tumor is located sub-capsularly or exophytically or surrounded by major vessels. The efficacy of RFA in HCC can be improved if combined with PEI. The combination of RFA and PEI was shown to be more effective than RFA alone for high-risk locations [15, 16].

In Cha et al. study, they tried to compare the efficacy and safety of PEI alone with PEI combined with RFA for HCCs in high-risk locations [15]. There were 20 HCCs (1.7±0.9 cm) in 20 patients (PEI group, $n=12$; PEI-RFA group, $n=8$). After treatment, technical success was achieved in all HCCs in both groups. During follow-up, local tumor progression was found in 41.7 % (5/12) in the PEI group, whereas 12.5 % (1/8) for the PEI+RFA group ($P=0.32$). Bile duct dilatation was the most common complication, especially when the tumors were in periportal locations, 55 % (5/9) in the PEI group and 50 % (2/4) in the PEI-RFA group ($P=1.00$). One patient in the PEI group developed severe biliary stricture and upstream dilatation that resulted in atrophy of the left hepatic lobe. One patient treated with PEI-RFA developed cholangitis and an abscess. They considered that combined PEI and RFA treatment has a tendency to be more effective than PEI alone for managing HCCs in high-risk locations, although the difference is not statistically significant. Even though PEI is generally accepted as a safe procedure, it may cause major biliary complications for managing HCCs adjacent to the portal vein.

Wong et al. conducted another study to investigate whether combining percutaneous PEI with RFA in the management of hepatocellular carcinoma (HCC) in high-risk locations improves treatment outcomes [16]. The study included 142 patients with 208 HCCs managed with radiofrequency ablation. Despite larger tumor sizes (2.8±1 cm vs. 1.9±0.7 cm vs. 2.5±0.1 cm for the high-risk radiofrequency plus PEI, non-high-risk radiofrequency, and high-risk radiofrequency groups, respectively; $P<0.001$), the primary effectiveness rate of high-risk radiofrequency ablation and PEI (92 %) was similar to that of non-high-risk radiofrequency ablation (96 %). The primary effectiveness rate of high-risk radiofrequency ablation and PEI was slightly higher ($P=0.1$) than that of high-risk radiofrequency ablation (85 %). The local tumor progression rates (21 % vs. 33 % vs. 24 % at 18 months) of the three respective groups were not statistically different ($P=0.91$). Patients with and those without high-risk tumors had equal survival rates ($P=0.42$) after 12 (87 % vs. 100 %) and 24 (77 % vs. 80 %) months of follow-up. Independent predictors of primary effectiveness were a tumor size of 3 cm or less ($P=0.01$) and distinct tumor borders ($P=0.009$). Indistinct borders ($P=0.033$) and nontreatment-naïve status of HCC ($P=0.002$) were associated with higher local tumor progression rates. The only predictor of survival was complete ablation of all index tumors ($P=0.001$). They considered that the combination of radiofrequency ablation and PEI in the management of HCC in high-risk locations has a slightly higher primary effectiveness rate than does radiofrequency ablation alone. But randomized controlled studies are warranted.

## 8.4 Combined with Surgical Treatment

Liver transplantation is an ideal cure therapy of HCC, better than surgical resection. Because liver transplantation removes not only the tumor-bearing liver, it also replaces the underlying cirrhotic liver with a normal liver and treats portal hypertension. But because of the deficiency of organ donor, some patients lose the opportunity of liver transplantation because of tumor regression during the waiting time. A study reported that 57 % of patients were rolled out during the waiting time without any treatment [17], so it is needed to reduce the dropout rate for the patients waiting for liver transplantation during waiting time. A clinical trial showed 50 patients with liver cirrhosis took RFA treatment before liver transplantation, 1- and 3-year survival rate was 95 % and 83 %, only two patients died of tumor recurrence, the major complication of patients with Child-Pugh B–C class was only 8 %, and this study indicated that it's effective and safe to slow down tumor regression by means of RFA [18]. Regarding the concern about the risk of seeding after RFA, it was only 0–1.4 % that has been confirmed in other recent studies [19]. RFA is a safe and promising bridge to liver transplantation.

Besides, RFA also can be used in surgical resection, especially patients with liver metastases which traditionally are assigned to be unresectable. Combined surgical resection and RFA is an effective and safe treatment modality for multifocal HCCs. Chio et al. reported 53 patients with 148 HCCs in their livers underwent surgical resection combined with ultrasound-guided intraoperative RFA, 1-, 3-, and 5-year survival rates were 87 %, 80 %, and 55 %, respectively, and there was one patient who suffered RFA-related complication [20]. But another study showed satellite lesions of non-resectable HCC took RFA treatment as adjuvant therapy, 3- and 5-year survival rates were 35.7 and 7.7 %, respectively, and they pointed out the existence of satellite lesions indicted that there was latent metastases that cannot be found and removed, so they believed taking RFA as adjuvant treatment was useless for HCC with satellite lesions [21]. But combined RFA with surgical resection can be an option of unresectable HCC. RFA also can be used as an instrument during operation because it can achieve liver coagulation necrosis, and radiofrequency-assisted liver resection (RF-R) can produce a "drying section" which can achieve minimal blood loss and reduce post-operation complication. Some studies showed the blood loss and rate of local recurrence were favorable. There also could be an oncologic benefit due to additional functional margin obtained with the RF effect. The 5-year recurrence rate of HCC resection is 77–100 %, 80–95 % of which is intrahepatic recurrence, and the first option for treating recurrence HCC is surgical resection. But only 10.4–27.4 % patients can receive surgical resection because of the characters of tumor, liver function, and the risk of surgery. Chio et al. evaluated the survival results and safety of RFA for recurrent HCC after hepatectomy; it turned out that 1-, 3-, and 5-year survival rates were 93.9, 65.7, and 51.6 %, respectively; and the cumulative rates of local tumor progression at 1, 3, and 5 years were 6.0, 8.6, and 11.9 % [22]. Liang et al. analyzed a cohort of 110 patients with recurrence of HCC. Sixty-six patients with 88 tumors were treated by RFA; 44 patients with 55 tumors were treated by repeat hepatectomy; 1-, 3-, and 5-year survival rates of RFA and repeat hepatectomy were 76.6, 48.6, and 39.9 and 78.6, 44.5, and 27.6 %; and there was no difference between RFA and hepatectomy treating recurrence HCC. Subgroup analyses showed that there was no significant difference for recurrent tumor ≤3 or >3 cm. But major complications happened more often after repeat hepatectomy than RFA [23]. With regard to treating recurrent HCC, RFA has showed advantages: minimally invasive, safe, more indications, and easily repeatable.

## 8.5 Combined with Sorafenib

Sorafenib, a tyrosine kinase inhibitor (TKI), has shown clinical efficacy in patients with HCC and is an important molecular-targeted drug for treating HCC. Sorafenib has become standard treatment of advanced HCC, and the median survival of patients with advanced HCC is nearly 3 months longer for patients treated with sorafenib than for those given placebo [24]. The effect and mechanism of RFA combined with sorafenib were studied firstly in animal model. Xu et al. conducted a study to evaluate the potential role of sorafenib as an adjunct to RFA to reduce the recurrence rate after insufficient RFA [25]. By comparing the control group with the RFA group, they found that insufficient RFA can promote HIF-1α and VEGFA expression ($P<0.05$). Similar results were also obtained for microvascular density (MVD) expression. Interestingly, by comparing to the RFA group, HIF-1α and VEGFA expression was significantly decreased in the group that received RFA combined with sorafenib treatment ($P<0.05$). Additionally, the combination of RFA with sorafenib therapy resulted in a synergistic reduction in tumor growth compared to insufficient RFA and sham puncture ($P<0.05$). The authors conclude that the combination of RFA with sorafenib resulted in reduced residual tumor volume due to reduced HIF-1a and VEGFA expression compared to RFA alone. Given the known mode of sorafenib activity and its inhibitory effects on the VEGFR and PDGFR signal pathways as well as the Ras-Raf-Erk pathway, this reduction of HIF-1a and VEGFA expression may be the mechanism that leads to the decreased tumor volume and reduced proliferation of HCC cells. Mertens et al. tried to investigate the effects of sorafenib when combined with RFA treatment in liver tissue, and the necrosis volume, tissue repair, and hepatocellular growth signals were analyzed in rats [26]. In that study, the authors showed in a rat model that the combination of RFA with the multi-tyrosine kinase inhibitor sorafenib results in a sustained necrosis volume due to reduced tissue repair compared to controls. And they thought that the mechanism leading to this promotion of necrosis is most probably a reduced proliferation of hepatocytes in the perinecrotic area and a reduced angiogenesis leading to a lack of microvessels in the zone of tissue repair. But in further observation, they found that the persistence of necrosis volume was a transient effect, despite the fact that sorafenib

was administered all through the post-RFA period. They found that hepatic growth factor (HGF) and epidermal growth factor (EGF) were significantly overexpressed in the sorafenib-treated animals. Interestingly, the described overexpression was also seen in areas of the liver distant from the immediate RFA damage indicating a generalized activation of proliferative signaling in the whole organ. Taken together, sorafenib-treated animals showed a transient delay in necrosis repair and at the same time an overexpression of proliferation-related genes (HGF and EGF) with a strong peak thereafter and a rapid decrease of overexpression thereafter. This supposedly results in a "growth spurt" with an accelerated tissue healing. Although the mechanism of combined sorafenib and RFA is not clear, some authors have investigated the role of combination in clinical trials.

Li's study assessed clinical efficacy and safety of sorafenib combined with TACE and RFA on patients with unresectable HCC. Efficacy and safety profiles of sorafenib in combination with TACE and RFA were evaluated based on retrospective data for 30 patients with unresectable HCC [27]. Patients were treated with TACE initially, followed by RFA 3 days after TACE. Seven days after the first TACE, patients started taking continuous sorafenib 400 mg bid without breaks until unacceptable toxicities or disease progression. The response to treatment, overall survival (OS), time to progression (TTP), and adverse effects were evaluated. The disease control rate was 33.3 % by RECIST criteria. The median TTP was 15.3 months (95 % CI 4.8–23.5). The median OS was 28.8 months (95 % CI 12.8–39.6). At the time of data record, 13 patients (43.3 %) were dead. Median OS in patients with or without portal vein thrombosis was 12.3 months (95 % CI 7.6–14.5) and 30.2 months (95 % CI 24.2–34.5), respectively ($P=0.018$). The most common adverse events related to sorafenib were hand-foot skin reaction (53.3 %) and diarrhea (33.3 %). The combination of sorafenib, TACE, and RFA proved both safe and effective in the treatment for unresectable hepatocellular carcinoma patients. The data of this study is exciting, but there is no direct evidence of efficacy and effect for sorafenib after curative treatment, such as RFA. A clinical trial to examine the recurrence-preventing effect of sorafenib by administration of it after curative treatment such as resection or ablation is in progress (STORM trial: http://clinicaltrials.gov.com, NCT00692770). This phase III randomized, double-blind, placebo-controlled study will evaluate the safety and efficacy of sorafenib versus placebo in patients with HCC after potential curative treatment (surgical resection or local ablation). The enrollment goal is 1100 patients. The primary outcome measure is recurrence-free survival, with secondary measure of time to disease recurrence, overall survival, patient-reported outcomes, and evaluation of biomarkers. Patients in this trial must have undergone surgical resections or local ablation for the treatment of HCC with curative intent within 4 months staging to potentially curative treatment. A maximum of two local ablation courses may be administered during this time period, and it should be 4 weeks ($28 \pm 7$ days) from the time of surgical resection or last local ablation course to the date of CT/magnetic resonance imaging scan. Patients should be free of original tumor. They should also have an intermediate or high risk of disease recurrence as assessed by tumor characteristics, a Child-Pugh score of 5–7 points, an Eastern Cooperation Oncology Group performance of 0, adequate bone marrow and live and renal function, and age older than 18 years, among other criteria. We hope the result of this trial. We also come up a theory that for the patients taking sorafenib, they can also take RFA as a palliative cytoreductive treatment, reducing the burden of tumor, to achieve a longer survival time. Until now, there are little relative studies on this point.

## 8.6 Combined with Chemotherapeutic Adjuvants

The intra-arterial administration of eluting doxorubicin on a bead has been demonstrated to enhance the effect of RFA for patients with medium to large HCC. RFA at a temperature lower than 50 °C induces reversible microvascular stasis and increases endothelial permeability and cytotoxicity of some chemotherapeutic agents. On the basis of this synergistic antineoplastic effect, it has been demonstrated that combined RFA and intravenous liposomal doxorubicin increases intratumoral accumulation of doxorubicin, increases coagulation necrosis, reduces tumor growth, and increases animal survival in rat breast tumor model studies. A pilot clinical study has also suggested that adjuvant liposomal doxorubicin chemotherapy increases tumor destruction, in contrast to RFA alone, in a variety of focal liver tumors. However, only one patient with HCC received combination therapy of liposomal doxorubicin and RFA in the study, and the synergistic antineoplastic effect for HCC may differ from that of liver metastasis. Recently, Wang et al. performed a trial to assess the therapeutic effect of a combination of hyperthermia therapy using RFA and intravenous chemotherapeutic agent for small HCC. Compared with RFA alone, Wang's study demonstrated that intravenous liposomal doxorubicin administration before RFA did not increase ablation volume for small HCC. Although there was significantly reduced contraction of ablative volume in the combination treatment group, liposomal doxorubicin administered intravenously before RFA had no impact on local recurrence, distant tumor progression, or patient's survival in follow-up [28]. However, in Hong's study, drug-plus-RFA combination therapy was used to completely treat an HCC in a patient who underwent liver transplantation 79 days later [29]. These differing results might be explained by differences in ablation protocol, tumor characteristics, and tumor size between these studies. However, the result of Wang's study has limitation due to the relatively small number of patients enrolled and low significance obtained. It might be too early to reach the conclusion that there is no synergistic effect of chemotherapeutic agents and RFA in delaying recurrence and prolonging survival for patients with small HCC. The synergistic effect might be affected by the dosage, timing of administration, circulation time, and administrative agents. Studies with more patients, uniform protocol, and long-term follow-up are necessary to clarify whether or not liposomal doxorubicin before RFA offered survival benefit for patients with HCC. Since completion of the phase I trial, a randomized phase III study comparing RFA plus drug with RFA plus placebo for HCC (search for NCT00617981 at http://clinicaltrials.gov/) has completed accrual, and data are being evaluated. The maximum tolerated dose of liposomal doxorubicin is 50 mg/m$^2$. This will be a phase III, randomized, double-blinded, dummy-controlled, efficacy, and safety study of liposomal doxorubicin plus RFA versus RFA plus dummy infusion. The 50 mg/m$^2$ liposomal doxorubicin or dummy infusion will be administered intravenously over 30 min. As part of blinded premedication, liposomal doxorubicin-treated subjects will receive 20 mg of dexamethasone orally 48 h prior to the drug infusion for infusion reaction prophylaxis. Subjects on the control arm will receive a matching dummy premedication pill orally at 48 h prior to infusion of the study treatment. Thirty minutes prior to receiving the liposomal doxorubicin infusion, subjects will receive a blinded dose of 20 mg of intravenous dexamethasone, 50 mg intravenous diphenhydramine, and either 50 mg of intravenous ranitidine or 20 mg of intravenous famotidine. Subjects on the control arm will receive a masked dummy premedication pill orally at 48 h prior to infusion of the study medication and a dummy infusion 30 min prior to dummy infusion of D5W (250 cc of 5 % dextrose solution). RFA will be initiated approximately at a minimum of 15 min after the initiation of study drug infusion and should be completed no later than 3 h after study of drug infusion initiation. The total length of the RFA procedure is proportional to the size of the tumor(s) involved and is anticipated to range from 12 to 60 min for each lesion with an estimated overall procedure time of less than 3 h. Subjects with incomplete ablations will be retreated to complete the ablation according to the treatment assigned at randomization. The completion of an ablation in this manner will restart the timeline of the study-related visits/procedures. This repeated ablation procedure cannot occur earlier than 21 days post-ablation but no later than 14 days after the first post-ablation CT

scan assessment. These subjects will start over at screening. If a complete ablation is not achieved after these two study treatments, the subject will be considered a treatment failure, and the patient will be discontinued and followed for survival only.

Subjects who recur with local and/or distant intrahepatic HCC after a complete initial ablation will have met the primary endpoint of progression-free survival. However, if these subjects have lesions that are amenable to RFA, the standard of care is to consider them for repeat RFA. Therefore, these subjects may receive treatment to which they were randomized if they continue to meet the inclusion and exclusion criteria of the protocol. Subjects who develop any extrahepatic lesion will have met the primary endpoint and will be discontinued from study treatment but will still be followed for overall survival. Dynamic contrast CT imaging will be used to assess the effectiveness of the ablation therapy. The blind will be maintained at the level of CT scan reads. All protocol-specified CT images will be centrally read and assessed by the endpoint committee in a blinded fashion. Posttreatment CT scans will be obtained at months 1, 3, 5, 7, 9, and 12 and every 3 months thereafter until withdrawal. Adverse event assessments and laboratory examinations will occur at each visit. All subjects will be monitored throughout the investigational period. Patients that meet inclusion/exclusion criteria may be at risk for contrast-induced nephropathy (CIN) when undergoing the required CT with contrast procedures. The investigators must be mindful of the risk factors (e.g., diabetes, borderline renal function) associated with CIN and employ strategies to reduce the risk of CIN. In subjects with diabetes or borderline renal function (creatinine greater than 1.5 mg/dL), special precautions (e.g., hydration, contrast dose reduction, follow-up creatinine determination) should be employed. An accepted procedure is adequate intravenous volume expansion with isotonic saline (1.0–1.5 mL/kg/h) for 3–12 h before the procedure and continued for 6–24 h. All randomized subjects will be followed for safety and overall survival.

## 8.7 Combined with Immune-Biological Treatment

The human immune system against the tumor is mainly dependent on the cellular immunity. Patients with HCC are found to have functional deficiency in a variety of immunocytes. Thus, cellular immunotherapy (CIT) would improve the immune state to afford a potential value in enhancing the therapeutic outcome for HCC patients. Current attempts at harnessing the immune system to eliminate tumors have been focusing on vaccination, such as dendritic cells (DCs) vaccine to increase the frequency of tumor-specific cytotoxic T lymphocytes (CTLs), and adoptive transfer of effector T cells and natural killer (NK) and γdT cells to promote tumor regression. The high temperature of RFA results in coagulation necrosis of HCC tissue, which not only breaks the body's immune suppression status by reducing the tumor burden but also increases the exposure of tumor cell epitopes and promotes the synthesis of heat shock protein (HSP) to effectively activate antitumor immune response. The cytokine and/or chemokine milieu might also enhance the antineoplastic function and promote the recruitment of circulating immune cells to the tumor site. Therefore, the CIT has been proposed for the patients with HCC to activate the immune function after RFA and may become an approach to effective control of recurrence and metastasis. There was a study that reported the combination of RFA and autologous RetroNectin activated killer (RAK) cells in the treatment of HCC patients with a tumor size less than 4 cm, and there are seven patients in analysis [30]. During a 7-month follow-up, no severe adverse events, recurrences, or deaths were observed in all seven HCC patients, the preliminary results suggested the feasibility and safety of the combined therapeutic regimen for HCC, and the RAK cell adoptive immunotherapy might be helpful in preventing recurrence in HCC patients after RFA. Due to the limited cases and follow-up visit period in this study, the long-term effects of combination treatment of RFA and RAK cells remain to be further validated, but this take a hope of another therapy to prevent HCC recurrence. By this study, the possibility for minimally invasive treatment combined with CIT using only one kind of immune cells has been explored with a reduction of short-term recurrence rate of HCC [30]. However, there are multiple mechanisms involved in the immune escape of the tumors. CIT with only one kind of immune cells is far to achieve the optimal immune escape of the tumors. In Cui's study, the synergistic effect of CIT with NK, γdT, and CIK cells was exploited [31]. In this study, the authors tried not only to administrate CIT at ideal time but also to apply the CIT with multiple kinds of cells to reach the optimal outcome. In this study, 62 patients with HCC who were treated with radical RFA were divided into two groups: RFA alone (32 patients) and RFA/CIT (30 patients). Autologous mononuclear cells were collected from the peripheral blood and separated by apheresis and then induced into natural killer (NK) cells, γdT cells, and cytokine-induced killer (CIK) cells. These cells were identified by flow cytometry with their specific antibodies and then were infused intravenously to RFA/CIT patients for three or six courses. The results implied that progression-free survival (PFS) was higher in RFA/CIT group than that in RFA group. In RFA/CIT group, six courses had better survival prognosis than three courses. Viral load of hepatitis C was decreased in two of three patients without antiviral therapy in RFA/CIT group but was increased in RFA group. No significant adverse reaction was found in the patients with CIT. Combination of sequential CIT with RFA for HCC patients was efficient and safe and may be helpful in the prevention of the recurrence for the patients with HCC after RFA. However, the relative small number of cases and the relative short follow-up periods reduced the importance of this study. Based on great advances in the understanding of the rules that guide immune activation against cancer, more and more studies confirmed that combination of conventional HCC therapy with immune stimulation appears to be a very promising approach. And the optimal immunotherapeutic strategies in HCC will presumably involve multiple immune effector mechanisms.

# References

1. Chen MS, Li JQ, Zheng YJ, et al. A prospective randomized trial comparing percutaneous local ablative therapy and partial hepatectomy for small hepatocellular carcinoma. Ann Surg. 2006;243:321–8.
2. Llovet JM, Burroughs A, Bruix J. Hepatocellular carcinoma. Lancet. 2003;362:1907–17.
3. Rossi S, Garbagnati F, Lencioni R, et al. Percutaneous radio-frequency thermal ablation of nonresectable hepatocellular carcinoma after occlusion of tumor blood supply. Radiology. 2000;217:119–26.
4. Seki T, Tamai T, Nakagawa T, et al. Combination therapy with transcatheter arterial chemoembolization and percutaneous microwave coagulation therapy for hepatocellular carcinoma. Cancer. 2000;89:1245–51.
5. Shibata T, Isoda H, Hirokawa Y, et al. Small hepatocellular carcinoma: is radiofrequency ablation combined with transcatheter arterial chemoembolization more effective than radiofrequency ablation alone for treatment? Radiology. 2009;252:905–13.
6. Morimoto M, Numata K, Kondou M, et al. Midterm outcomes in patients with intermediate-sized hepatocellular carcinoma: a randomized controlled trial for determining the efficacy of radiofrequency ablation combined with transcatheter arterial chemoembolization. Cancer. 2010;116:5452–60.
7. Peng ZW, Zhang YJ, Chen MS, et al. Radiofrequency ablation with or without transcatheter arterial chemoembolization in the treatment of hepatocellular carcinoma: a prospective randomized trial. J Clin Oncol. 2013;31:426–32.
8. Yang W, Chen MH, Wang MQ, et al. Combination therapy of radiofrequency ablation and transarterial chemoembolization in recurrent hepatocellular carcinoma after hepatectomy compared with single treatment. Hepatol Res. 2009;39:231–40.
9. Shen SQ, Xiang JJ, Xiong CL, et al. Intraoperative radiofrequency thermal ablation combined with portal vein infusion chemotherapy and transarterial chemoembolization for unresectable HCC. Hepatogastroenterology. 2005;52:1403–7.
10. Yan S, Xu D, Sun B. Combination of radiofrequency ablation with transarterial chemoembolization for hepatocellular carcinoma: a meta-analysis. Dig Dis Sci. 2012;57:3026–31.
11. Wang W, Shi J, Xie WF. Transarterial chemoembolization in combination with percutaneous ablation therapy in unresectable hepatocellular carcinoma: a meta-analysis. Liver Int. 2010;30:741–9.
12. Schwartz M, Weintraub J. Combined transarterial chemoembolization and radiofrequency ablation for hepatocellular carcinoma. Nat Clin Pract Oncol. 2008;5:630–1.
13. Peng ZW, Zhang YJ, Chen MS, et al. Recurrent hepatocellular carcinoma treated with sequential transcatheter arterial chemoembolization and radiofrequency ablation versus radiofrequency abla-

tion alone: a prospective randomized trial. Radiology. 2012;262:689–700.
14. Zhang YJ, Liang HH, Chen MS, et al. Hepatocellular carcinoma treated with radiofrequency ablation with or without ethanol injection: a prospective randomized trial. Radiology. 2007;244:599–607.
15. Cha DI, Lee MW, Rhim H, et al. Therapeutic efficacy and safety of percutaneous ethanol injection with or without combined radiofrequency ablation for hepatocellular carcinomas in high risk locations. Korean J Radiol. 2013;14:240–7.
16. Wong SN, Lin CJ, Lin CC, Chen WT, Cua IH, Lin SM. Combined percutaneous radiofrequency ablation and ethanol injection for hepatocellular carcinoma in high-risk locations. AJR Am J Roentgenol. 2008;190:W187–95.
17. Fisher RA, Maluf D, Cotterell AH, et al. Non-resective ablation therapy for hepatocellular carcinoma: effectiveness measured by intention-to-treat and dropout from liver transplant waiting list. Clin Transplant. 2004;18:502–12.
18. Mazzaferro V, Battiston C, Perrone S, et al. Radiofrequency ablation of small hepatocellular carcinoma in cirrhotic patients awaiting liver transplantation: a prospective study. Ann Surg. 2004;240:900–9.
19. Latteri F, Sandonato L, Di Marco V, et al. Seeding after radiofrequency ablation of hepatocellular carcinoma in patients with cirrhosis: a prospective study. Dig Liver Dis. 2008;40:684–9.
20. Choi D, Lim HK, Joh JW, et al. Combined hepatectomy and radiofrequency ablation for multifocal hepatocellular carcinomas: long-term follow-up results and prognostic factors. Ann Surg Oncol. 2007;14:3510–8.
21. Taniai N, Yoshida H, Mamada Y, et al. Is intraoperative adjuvant therapy effective for satellite lesions in patients undergoing reduction surgery for advanced hepatocellular carcinoma? Hepatogastroenterology. 2006;53(68):258–61.
22. Choi D, Lim HK, Rhim H, et al. Percutaneous radiofrequency ablation for recurrent hepatocellular carcinoma after hepatectomy: long-term results and prognostic factors. Ann Surg Oncol. 2007;14:2319–29.
23. Liang HH, Chen MS, Peng ZW, et al. Percutaneous radiofrequency ablation versus repeat hepatectomy for recurrent hepatocellular carcinoma: a retrospective study. Ann Surg Oncol. 2008;15:3484–93.
24. Llovet JM, Ricci S, Mazzaferro V, et al. Sorafenib in advanced hepatocellular carcinoma. N Engl J Med. 2008;359:378–90.
25. Xu M, Xie XH, Xie XY, et al. Sorafenib suppresses the rapid progress of hepatocellular carcinoma after insufficient radiofrequency ablation therapy: an experiment in vivo. Acta Radiol. 2013;54:199–204.
26. Mertens JC, Martin IV, Schmitt J, et al. Multikinase inhibitor sorafenib transiently promotes necrosis after radiofrequency ablation in rat liver but activates growth signals. Eur J Radiol. 2012;81:1601–6.

27. Li Y, Zheng YB, Zhao W, et al. Sorafenib in combination with transarterial chemoembolization and radiofrequency ablation in the treatment for unresectable hepatocellular carcinoma. Med Oncol. 2013;30:730.

28. Goldberg SN, Kamel JR, Kruskal JB, et al. Radiofrequency ablation of hepatic tumors: increased tumor destruction with adjuvant liposomal doxorubicin therapy. Am J Roentgenol. 2002;179:93–101.

29. Wang JH, Tung HD, Chen TY, et al. Radiofrequency ablation of small hepatocellular carcinoma with intravenous pegylated liposomal doxorubicin. Hepatol Int. 2010;5:567–74.

30. Hong CW, Libutti SK, Wood BJ. Liposomal doxorubicin plus radiofrequency ablation for complete necrosis of a hepatocellular carcinoma. Curr Oncol. 2013;20:e274–7.

31. Ma HQ, Zhang YJ, Wang QJ, et al. Therapeutic safety and effects of adjuvant autologous RetroNectin activated killer cell immunotherapy for patients with primary hepatocellular carcinoma after radiofrequency ablation. Cancer Biol Ther. 2010;9:903–7.

# Radiological Assessment and Follow-Up After Radiofrequency Ablation

Ming Kuang

## 9.1 Follow-Up

Close and regular follow-up is recommended for patients following radiofrequency ablation (RFA) [1]. Baseline ultrasound (US) examinations should be performed within 24 h after ablation to exclude complications. Contrast-enhanced imaging can be performed within 24 h for early evaluation of therapeutic responses or possible complications (e.g., residual tumor tissue) [2]. During follow-up, the effectiveness of RFA should also be assessed by imaging 1 month after treatment to assess the inflammation surrounding the ablation zone. Appropriate imaging modalities could be contrast-enhanced US (ceUS), contrast-enhanced computed tomography (ceCT), or contrast-enhanced magnetic resonance imaging (ceMRI). Liver function and serum α-fetoprotein (AFP) should also be measured in the first month after ablation. The combination of laboratory tests and imaging examinations can make definite assessments. Contrast-enhanced imaging should determine whether the tumor was entirely covered by the ablation zone, whether new HCC lesions have occurred, and whether any normal adjacent

structures were affected during ablation. Tumors without enhancement in the ablation zone are considered completely ablated, and if any enhancement is observed, tumors should be considered incompletely ablated. A recurrent hepatic tumor can be classified as local tumor progress (LTP) or a distal intrahepatic recurrence. LTP is defined as a recurrent tumor that occurs inside or adjacent to the primary tumor volume following a complete ablation. Distal intrahepatic recurrences are defined as intrahepatic lesions that are separated from the ablation zone by more than 1 cm. Distant recurrences can include intrahepatic recurrences and extrahepatic metastases. RFA effectiveness should be assessed according to whether the technique was successfully implemented. Technical success is defined when the tumor was treated according to protocol and was completely covered by the ablation zone. Otherwise, the treatment is defined as a technical failure. Technique effectiveness refers to complete ablation of a macroscopic tumor at a prospectively defined time point (frequently 1 month post-treatment). For cases of complete ablation and no recurrence at 1 month post-treatment, follow-ups should include abdominal US, serum AFP, and liver function measurements. They should be performed every month for 3 months, then every 3 months until 2 years post-treatment. After 2 years post-treatment, follow-ups should be performed every 6 months. Contrast-enhanced

M. Kuang, MD, PhD
Department of Hepatobiliary Surgery, The First
Affiliated Hospital of Sun Yat-sen University,
Guangzhou, China
e-mail: kuangm@mail.sysu.edu.cn

© Springer Science+Business Media Dordrecht 2016
M. Chen et al. (eds.), *Radiofrequency Ablation for Small Hepatocellular Carcinoma*,
DOI 10.1007/978-94-017-7258-7_9

imaging should be performed to confirm the diagnosis of suspicious lesions that are detected upon abdominal US or if serum AFP levels become elevated again. ceCT or ceMRI should be repeated every 6–12 months during follow-up [3].

## 9.2 Radiological Assessment

The accuracy of radiological imaging is rapidly evolving, and it can be used to assess the therapeutic efficacy of RFA by monitoring the dynamic evolution of the ablation zone and surrounding liver tissue and detect ablation-related complications and recurrences. US, including ceUS, ceCT, and ceMRI, is commonly used for RFA follow-up [4]. Fluorine-18 fluorodeoxyglucose (FDG) positron emission tomography/computed tomography ($^{18}$F-FDG PET/CT) is occasionally required if there are difficulties in making diagnoses with other imaging modalities, and it can play an important role in assessing RFA treatment responses [5]. Imaging changes that are observed in the liver after RFA of HCC can be broadly divided into normal changes, residual tumor, tumor recurrence, or complications [6–8].

## 9.3 Normal Changes

### 9.3.1 Ablation Zone

Patients undergo contrast-enhanced imaging examinations 1 month after RFA in most hospitals to assess the therapeutic efficacy. The ablation zone is roughly circular depending on the number of ablations and type of electrode. Multi-needle and -point ablations, or ablation zones adjacent to blood vessels, can lead to irregular shapes. With time, the ablation zones can shrink (Fig. 9.1) and borders become increasingly clear. Additionally, echogenicity upon US, density upon CT, and signal intensity upon MRI become more uniform. Shrinkage of the liver capsule is sometimes visible when the ablation zone is located in the subcapsular area. Compared to the volume immediately after RFA, the mean volume of ablation zones decreases to 79 % at 1 month, 50 % at 4 months, 27 % at 16 months, and 11 % at 19 months. Expansion of the ablation zone does not occur unless there are complications (such as biloma or hepatic abscess) or a tumor recurrence. In these situations, additional examination is warranted.

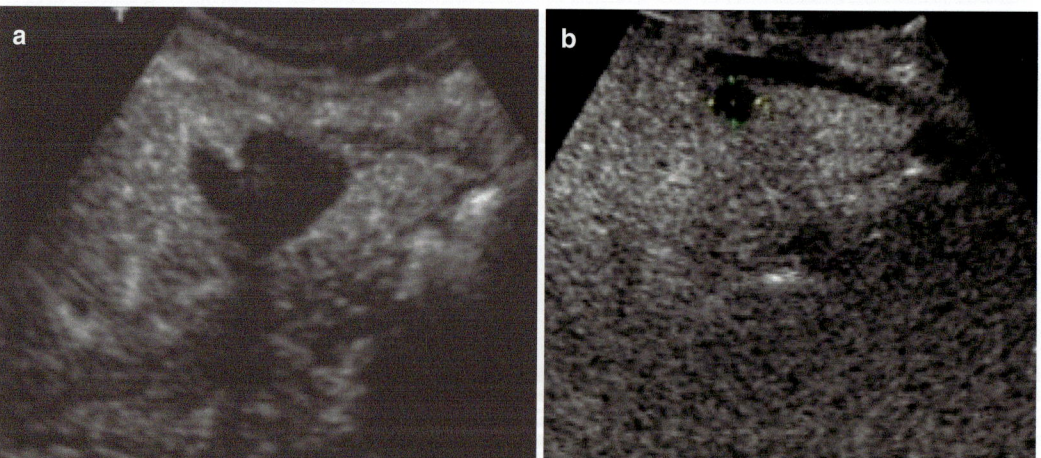

**Fig. 9.1** (**a**) Contrast-enhanced ultrasound image obtained 1 month after percutaneous RFA shows complete non-enhancement of the ablation zone. The ablation zone is irregular because of the location in the subcapsular area and adjacent to the blood vessels. (**b**) Contrast-enhanced ultrasound image obtained 42 months after ablation shows that the ablation zone has reduced in size

### 9.3.1.1 US and ceUS

Transient hyperechoic zones momentarily appear within and around a tumor on the baseline US both during and immediately after RFA due to gas bubble formation from water vaporization and necrosis of the tumor and liver tissue. The transient hyperechoic zone can persist for 30–90 min and can be used to roughly estimate the ablation zone during RFA. When the gas dissipates, the echogenicity of the ablation zone is heterogeneous, containing iso-echoic and hyperechoic regions. ceUS can be used after the disappearance of the transient hyperechoic zones to detect residual tumor if an incomplete ablation is suspected. One month after ablation, completely ablated, necrotic tumors appear as well-defined regions with heterogeneous echogenicity and no posterior acoustic enhancement. The ablation zone gradually becomes iso-echoic with time. The ablation zone must be larger than the original tumor, and the former will gradually shrink rather than expand. Sometimes, a hyperechoic needle tract is visible in the middle of or in front of the ablation zone. No internal flow can be visualized in the ablation zone upon Doppler US imaging. The ablation zone will show normal uptake and wash out of contrast agent signal throughout the three phases of CEUS, which are the arterial enhancement phase, portal venous enhancement phase, and interstitial enhancement or delayed phase. Contrast agents increase the accuracy of US, and the ablation zone should be measured using ceUS rather than the baseline ultrasound.

### 9.3.1.2 ceCT

CT without contrast agents, performed immediately after RFA, reveals a primarily low-density ablation zone. High-density regions representing intratumor bleeding or tissue dehydration can be seen in a few ablation zones. Additionally, small amounts of gas generated by tissue necrosis or boiling during RFA can be observed by CT. These air bubbles are usually round, tubular, or oval shaped and should not be mistaken for infection or a hepatic abscess caused by RFA. With time, the ablation zone evolves into a more homogeneous region of low density upon CT without contrast agents. Occasionally, the differences in tissue properties between the tumor and adjacent liver parenchyma create a target appearance of an ablation zone. A target appearance of an ablation zone is low density upon CT within the ablated tumor (presumably with prominent fatty metamorphosis) and is surrounded by a relatively high-density region of ablated liver parenchyma. The low density of ablated tumors may be due to fatty metamorphosis of HCC, and the high density of the ablated liver parenchyma helps to visualize the ablation margin. The electrode needle tract is often visible along the path of the RF electrode shaft in the ablation zone. It appears as a high-density charring shadow, which disappears over time. The ablation zone does not enhance during any phase of ceCT due to perfusion deficiencies. No expansion of unenhanced area is observed during the portal and delay phase [9].

### 9.3.1.3 ceMRI

One month after RFA, ablation zones display heterogeneous high-intensity signal upon T1-weighted MRI and either a homogeneous or heterogeneous low-intensity signal upon T2-weighted MRI without contrast enhancement. As time passes, the signal intensity of the ablation zone will gradually become higher on T1-weighted images and more homogeneously low upon T2-weighted imaging. The target appearance can also occur with MR imaging [10].

### 9.3.2 Transient Hyperemia Surrounding the Ablation Zone

Transient periablational hyperemia appears immediately after RFA in most cases. Liver tissue surrounding the necrotic ablation zone develops hyperemia and edema because of the thermal damage. Pathology has further revealed inflammation in blood vessels and the formation of granulation tissue. Transient periablational hyperemia usually disappears by 1 month post-ablation but can exist for up to 6 months.

Transient periablational hyperemia is hypo-echoic upon US, is low-density upon CT, and has a rim of slightly increased signal intensity upon T2-weighted MRI (Fig. 9.2). However, the hyperemia is usually subtle or nonexistent upon unenhanced imaging for most cases. After administration of contrast agents, transient hyperemia is clearly visualized as a thin (usually <5 mm) and uniform rim surrounding the abla-tion zone. It is hyperenhanced during the arterial phase and iso-enhanced during the portal and delay phases. This hyperemic rim should not be considered a residual tumor or tumor recurrence (Fig. 9.3).

### 9.3.3 Arterioportal Shunting

Arterioportal shunting is a common finding upon contrast-enhanced radiological imaging. It is due to mechanical or thermal injury of small hepatic vessels and results in abnormal perfusion to liver tissue that is adjacent to the ablation zone. Arterioportal shunting is visualized as a hyperen-hanced wedge shape during the arterial phase that is iso-enhanced during the portal and delayed phases. It is usually not observed upon imaging (US, CT, or MRI) without contrast enhancement. Arterioportal shunting will gradually resolve spontaneously [11].

## 9.4 Residual Tumors and Tumor Recurrence

### 9.4.1 Residual Tumors

Residual tumors occur when the ablation zone does not fully cover the HCC lesion. Residual tumors are always difficult to observe during baseline US or unenhanced CT, and they can occur as nodular lesions adjacent to the ablation zone. T2-weighted MRI can distinguish residual tumors. Residual tumors appear as nodular-like regions of high signal intensity residing next to the ablation margin or create irregular peripheral rims of high signal intensity that readily contrast against the low signal intensity background of the ablation zone. Upon contrast-enhanced radiological imaging, residual tumors appear as nodular or irregular hyperenhancements on the periphery of the ablation zone during the arterial phase that wash out during the portal or delay phase [12, 13].

[18]F-FDG PET/CT can play an important role in the assessment of the presence of residual tumors after RFA [5, 14]. The ablation zone appears cold upon PET imaging, while residual tumors appear as hot foci, indicating increased FDG uptake, adjacent to the ablation zone. Post-RFA inflammation around the ablation zone may also cause the increased FDG uptake. It appears

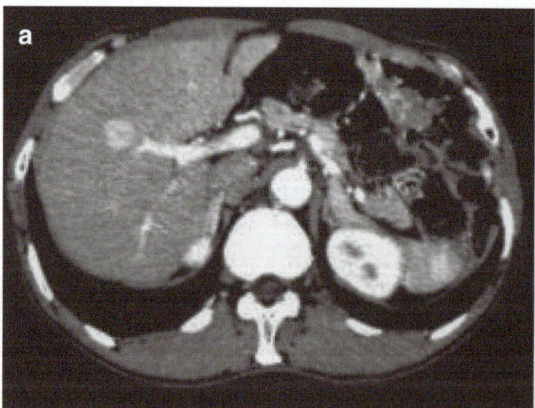
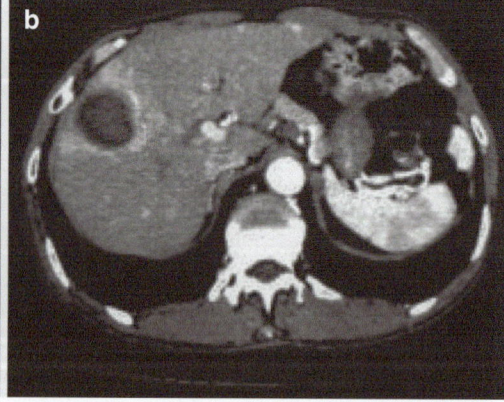
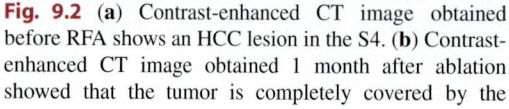

**Fig. 9.2** (a) Contrast-enhanced CT image obtained before RFA shows an HCC lesion in the S4. (b) Contrast-enhanced CT image obtained 1 month after ablation showed that the tumor is completely covered by the ablation zone. The RFA zone is round and surrounded by a thin and uniform contrast-enhanced rim, which repre-sents transient periablational hyperemia. Arterioportal shunting adjacent to the ablation zone is also depicted

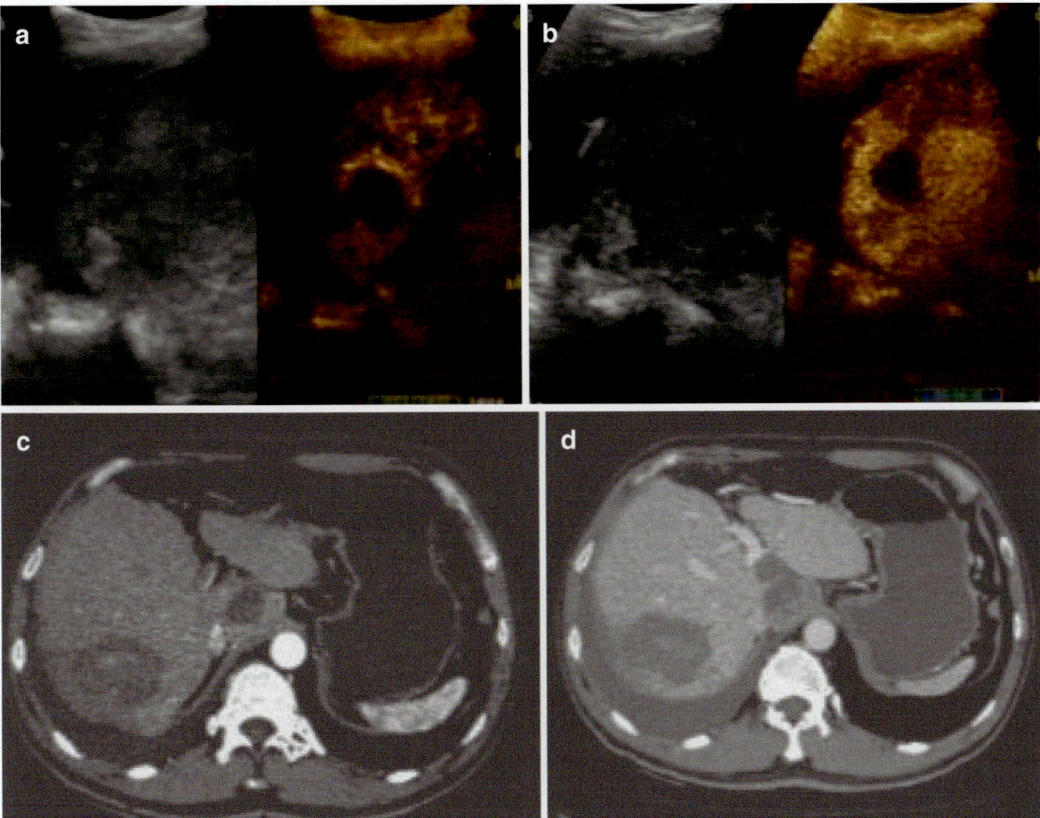

**Fig. 9.3** (**a**) The arterial phase of a follow-up contrast-enhanced ultrasound image in a 47-year-old male showed a thin and uniform contrast-enhanced rim surrounding the ablation zone and a nodular hyperenhancement on the posterior area of the ablation zone. These represent a transient periablational hyperemia and residual tumor, respectively. (**b**) Contrast-enhanced ultrasound image in the portal phase showed no wash out in the transient periablational hyperemia, but wash out in the residual tumor. Contrast-enhanced CT in the arterial phase (**c**) demonstrated the same nodular hyperenhancement and wash out in the portal phase (**d**)

as a low-grade homogeneous distribution of FDG signal surrounding the ablation zone. Residual tumors can be easily masked by this feature. FDG uptake associated with the post-RFA inflammation can appear as early as 2 or 3 days after RFA; hence, [18]F-FDG PET/CT examinations should be performed within 1–2 days after the ablation to detect residual tumor tissue.

### 9.4.2 Local Tumor Progress

LTP usually progresses beyond the ablation zone but initiates within it. Sometimes, LTP may occur through the entire ablation zone. When LTP is present, hypo-echoic nodular lesions will appear at the margin of the hyperechoic ablation zone upon baseline US. LTP has low density on unenhanced CT, low homogeneous signal intensity upon T1-weighted MRI, and slightly increased signal intensity upon T2-weighted MRI. After injection of contrast agents, LTP imaging findings are similar to those of small HCC lesions. If the tumor lacks adequate perfusion, LTP may manifest as an enlarged ablation zone or an uneven edge of the ablation zone, with irregular and less distinct margins. Intrahepatic recurrences and distant recurrences appear similar to HCC. 18F-FDG PET/CT imaging can also be used as an important method to detect tumor recurrences early. Tumor recurrences appear as foci of increased FDG uptake within or outside the ablation zone (Fig. 9.4) [14].

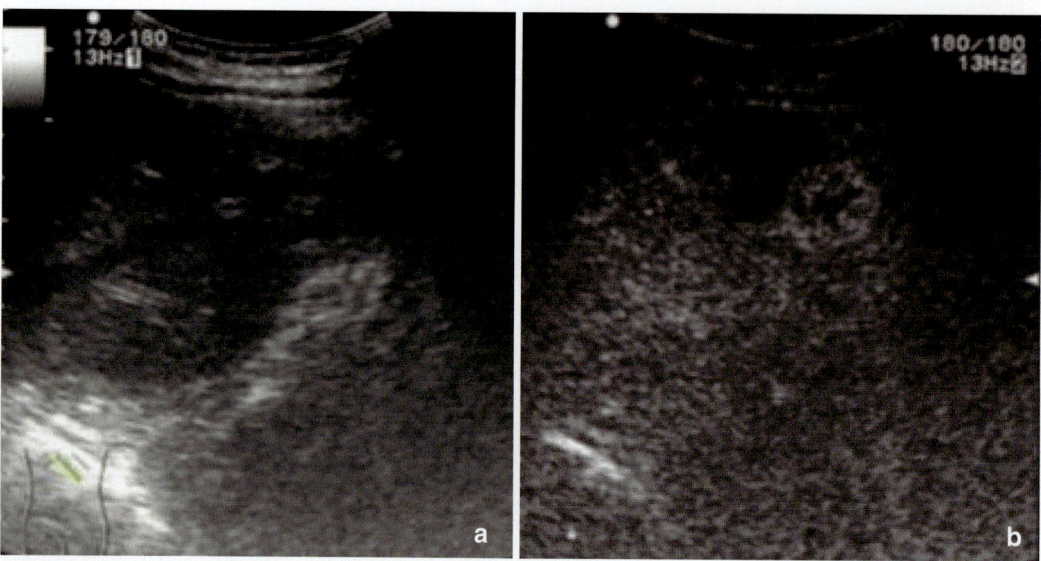

**Fig. 9.4** Baseline ultrasound image (**a**) of a 58-year-old male 6 months after ablation does not detect the nodular hyperenhancement during the arterial phase of contrast-enhanced ultrasound (**b**)

### 9.4.3 Residual Tumors and LTP

Residual tumors and LTP can be distinguished by transient hyperemia after ablation. The key features that differentiate them are whether the rim enhancement in the arterial phase is regular and uniform and whether the enhancement washes out in the portal or delayed phases. Additionally, detailed comparisons between preoperative and postoperative images and attentive follow-up care are essential to correctly distinguish each.

## 9.5 Complications

### 9.5.1 Vascular Complications

The most common vascular complication is bleeding. Bleeding appears as ascites, the number of which correlate with the quantity blood that enters the peritoneal cavity. A small amount of bleeding can gradually resolve spontaneously. Acute bleeding appears anechoic upon baseline US and as a low-density area upon unenhanced CT. A hepatic hematoma appears as a high-density feature in the acute phase, but the signal intensity of the blood changes over time. ceUS

can reveal bleeding by the leakage of US contrast agent into the peritoneal cavity [15].

A hepatic arterial pseudoaneurysm is another vascular complication. It is rare and thought to be caused by mechanical or thermal injury. This pseudoaneurysm appears as a round or oval anechoic area inside the ablation zone and possesses an arterial blood flow signal upon Doppler US. Upon unenhanced CT, pseudoaneurysms appear as fluid areas with high density. A hyperenhancement resembling the hepatic artery will appear during the arterial phase upon ceUS, ceCT, or ceMRI.

### 9.5.2 Bile Duct Complications

The main bile duct complications are bile duct dilatation and biloma. Bile duct dilatation often occurs in the bile duct surrounding the ablation zone or the distal bile duct adjacent to the ablation zone. It often resolves over time.

Bilomas occur most frequently in patients undergoing repeated ablations and always develops 2–4 months after ablation. However, it is occasionally found immediately after RFA. In most cases, bilomas are a minor complication of no clinical significance. They often appear as well-defined unilobular cystic masses with mural nodules and have crescent, round, or irregular shapes. Crescent bilomas are most common after RFA. Follow-up radiological images with enlargement of the ablation zone may suggest a biloma [16]. Cystic components of bilomas represent the bile and are anechoic upon baseline US and have low CT density without contrast enhancement. Most bilomas appear as low-density features with an attenuation <20 HU upon unenhanced CT. However, the attenuation of some bilomas can be >20 HU when hemorrhage, inflammatory cells, or necrotic debris is present. The mural nodules of bilomas represent the ablated tumor tissue and/or liver parenchyma. They are iso-echoic or slightly hyper-echoic upon baseline US and are isodense or hyperdense upon CT. Mural nodules remain unenhanced throughout all phases of contrast-enhanced imaging (Fig. 9.5).

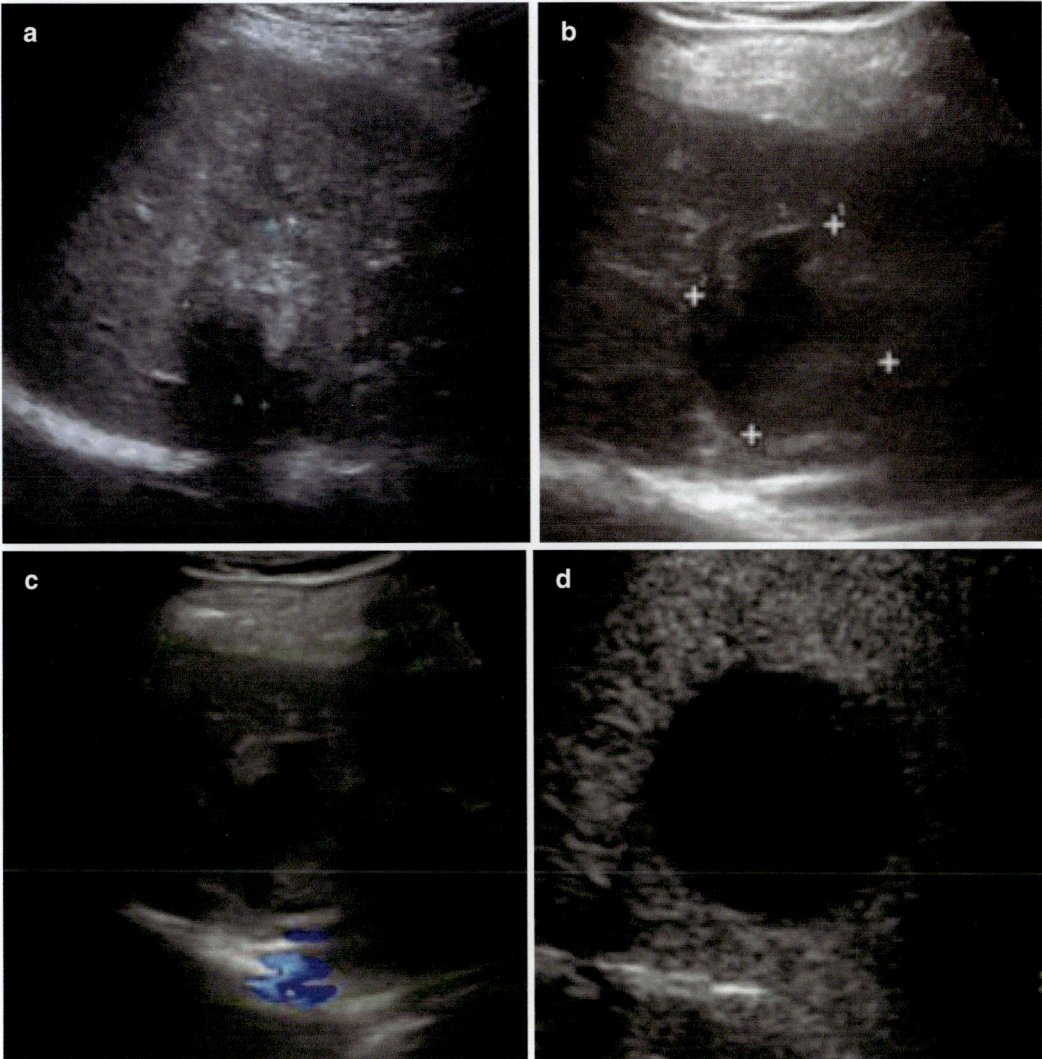

**Fig. 9.5** (**a**) Baseline ultrasound image 1 month after ablation shows a heterogeneous lesion without fluid-filled areas, which represents an ablation zone. (**b**) Baseline ultrasound image 3 months after ablation shows a heterogeneous cystic lesion with fluid-filled areas and a mural nodule, which represents the formation of a biloma. (**c**) No blood flow signal is detected in the mural nodules upon Doppler ultrasound imaging. (**d**) Contrast-enhanced ultrasound shows complete non-enhancement of the biloma

### 9.5.3 Infection

The most common result of infections in the liver is an abscess. Formation of a liver abscess takes several weeks. Abscesses occur in patients with the typical clinical symptoms, including fever and chills, malaise, abdominal pain, elevated white blood cell counts, and other clinical features. Enlargement of the ablation zone may suggest a hepatic abscess in patients with typical symptoms. Significant risk factors for liver abscess after RFA include preexisting biliary abnormalities which leave patients prone to ascending biliary infections, tumors that retain iodized oil, and using internally cooled electrodes. Abscesses that develop in the ablation zone are similar to other typical abscesses. A hepatic abscess typically presents as ill-defined, heterogeneous, cystic lesion with a thick wall, central fluid-filled areas with liquefaction, and posterior acoustic enhancement. They often contain septa, debris, and sometimes gas inside the lesion. They are hypo-echoic and have few internal flow signals upon Doppler US. They have low CT density upon ceCT, low signal intensity upon T1-weighted MRI, and high signal intensity upon T2-weighted MRI. During the three phases of contrast-enhanced imaging, they show thick, rim-like or honeycomb-like enhancement during the arterial phase with or without hyperenhanced liver tissue adjacent to the lesion. They have hypo-enhancement during the portal and late phases [17]. The gas inside hepatic abscesses, which mostly appeared as bubbles, is prominent and should not be mistaken as normal accumulation of gas that occurs after ablation. The appearance of gas bubbles can increase at later follow-up time points. Microbubbles produced by radiofrequency ablation are known to persist for 30–90 min after RFA. Hepatic abscesses should be strongly suspected when substantial air echogenicity is detected upon US at 1 day or later post-RFA. Detecting no air bubbles inside the ablation zone upon immediate follow-up imaging does not exclude subsequent infection of the ablation zone entirely. Gas bubbles can be observed later (e.g., 30 days after ablation) and suggest an abscess. Sometimes, the air-fluid ratio inside abscesses or a wedge-shaped perfusion defect (possible infarct) in the periphery of the ablation zone can be noted in the radiological findings. Cholangitis is a rare complication after the RFA. The major risk factors of cholangitis include cholangioenterostomy, biliary stent placement, hepatic artery chemoembolization, and diabetes. A radiological manifestation of cholangitis is the thickening of the bile duct wall during contrast-enhanced imaging [18].

### 9.5.4 Tumor Seeding

Tumor seeding in the needle tract is a rare complication after RFA. Contrast-enhanced imaging shows an irregularly enhanced tumor lesion along the needle tract that is similar to HCC. It should be distinguished from postoperative inflammation, and radiological follow-up or biopsy should be performed.

## 9.6 Advantages and Disadvantages of Radiological Imaging Modalities

The evaluation of RFA effectiveness for HCC is essential to devise further treatment and follow-up strategies. Evaluations are usually performed with US, CT, or MRI [19–25]. Conventional US is easy performed, repeatable, and inexpensive. It provides information about changes in the size, boundary, and echogenicity of the ablation zone. It can also reveal intrahepatic local and distant recurrences. Doppler US assesses blood flow in the ablation zone and adjacent liver tissue and whether flow is arterial or venous. It facilitates the evaluation of residual tumors and recurrences. However, due to the similar appearance of necrotic tissue and tumor tissue, conventional US lacks the necessary sensitivity and specificity for accurate diagnoses. Furthermore, the poor sensitivity of Doppler US to detect slow flow in small vessels surrounding the ablation zone limits the ability to detect residual tumors and recurrences. US has difficulty in determining whether tumors are necrotic or not [22].

Contrast-enhanced US with a low mechanical index allows dynamic real-time evaluation of both the macro- and micro-circulation of focal liver lesions throughout vascular phases and is superior to conventional ultrasound. ceUS can detect blood flow in small vessels [21]. ceUS is comparable to ceCT for evaluating tumor microcirculation. It is superior to ceCT for detecting tumor vasculature and imaging small lesions. ceUS can more sensitively evaluate efficacy because of real-time continuous dynamic observation. ceUS is also easy to perform, and therapeutic efficacy can be evaluated immediately by ceUS, which allows additional ablation if needed. Furthermore, ceUS using the contrast agent Levovist revealed more lesions than baseline ultrasound in 56 % of patients and more lesions than CT in 22 % patients during the delay phase [24]. However, ceUS also has significant drawbacks. First, ceUS has lower sensitivity to image the macro- and micro-circulation in tumors with minimal perfusion prior to ablation, which can affect the accuracy of evaluating therapy efficacy. Second, during ceUS imaging, radiologists only image part of the ablation zone and overlook residual or recurrent tumors, because ceUS is an operator-dependent imaging technology. Third, the ability of ceUS is affected by the tumor location, such as the anterior superficial or deep liver areas, and acoustic window. ceUS detection of hepatic lesions can be challenging in patients with lesions covered by the lung or diaphragm and in patients with obesity, meteorism, or cirrhosis.

ceCT and ceMRI are reliable and accurate imaging modalities to determine post-treatment efficacy and plan follow-up strategies. Both provide more information compared with the ultrasound and have become the most common methods to evaluate RFA efficacy. They have also replaced CT hepatic angiography. Three-dimensional CT or MRI can be used to assess the safety ablation margin. However, ceCT has a high rate of false-negatives when detecting small lesions and could easily lead to misdiagnoses. The sensitivity of postoperative CT to detect residual tumors within 24 h after RFA is only 20 %, which is lower than ceUS. When HCC is treated with TACE before RFA, ceCT may overestimate tumor response because lipiodol is retained inside the HCC nodules. Additionally, ceCT is unsuitable for patients with renal disease or allergies to contrast agents.

MRI has excellent resolution and sensitivity (up to 89 %) to detect residual tumors. It is widely used in the postoperative evaluations of RFA. MRI after RFA is more sensitive than CT, which is especially important to detect small lesions. MRI is more accurate than CT for measuring the size of the ablation zone. The error for MRI measurements is less than 2 mm when compared to histopathology. Diffusion-weighted imaging (DWI) sequences can identify small HCC lesions that can be difficult to detect using conventional MRI, and DWI can be used for early assessment of residual tumors or tumor recurrence. Tumors show high signal intensity on DWI, and when combined with conventional MRI, DWI improves diagnostic accuracy. The drawback of MRI is that it is expensive, time consuming, and cannot be used in patients with pacemakers or other ferromagnetic materials or those suffering from claustrophobia [19].

Unlike morphologic imaging modalities such as ultrasonography, CT, and MRI, [18]F-FDG PET/CT is a functional imaging modality. Hepatocellular carcinomas, including tumors of higher histologic grades, are associated with increased FDG uptake, and therefore, [18]F-FDG PET/CT could be used to assess the treatment response after the ablation of HCC lesions. [18F-FDG] PET/CT can detect changes in metabolism that reflect treatment responses sooner than morphologic imaging modalities. Therefore, it is used to assess treatment responses early in the course of RFA. [18]F-FDG PET/CT should be performed before inflammation and tissue regeneration processes at the periphery of the ablation zone begin. [18]F-FDG PET/CT cannot be used for regular examination during follow-up, and its use to measure RFA responses has been studied more extensively in metastatic liver tumors than in primary liver tumors [25].

## Conclusion

Radiological imaging is an important tool to assess the therapeutic efficacy of RFA in HCC. No residual or recurrent tumor after a comprehensive radiological examination and negative serum tumor markers can be used as a standard of clinical cure. Combining multiple imaging modalities to monitor post-ablation status is important to increase patient survival by assessing therapeutic efficacy and detecting residual or recurrent tumors.

## References

1. Llovet JM, Bruix J. Novel advancements in the management of hepatocellular carcinoma in 2008. J Hepatol. 2008;48 Suppl 1:S20–37.
2. Gallotti A, D'onofrio M, Ruzzenente A, et al. Contrast-enhanced ultrasonography (CEUS) immediately after percutaneous ablation of hepatocellular carcinoma. Radiol Med. 2009;114:1094–105.
3. Goldberg SN, Grassi CJ, Cardella JF, et al. Image-guided tumor ablation: standardization of terminology and reporting criteria. Radiology. 2005;235:728–39.
4. Kim SK, Lim HK, Kim YH, et al. Hepatocellular carcinoma treated with radiofrequency ablation: spectrum of imaging findings. Radiographics. 2003;23:107–21.
5. Nielsen K, van Tilborg AA, Scheffer HJ, et al. PET-CT after radiofrequency ablation of colorectal liver metastases: suggestions for timing and image interpretation. Eur J Radiol. 2013;82:2169–75.
6. Kim YS, Rhim H, Lim HK, et al. Coagulation necrosis induced by radiofrequency ablation in the liver: histopathologic and radiologic review of usual to extremely rare changes. Radiographics. 2011;31:377–90.
7. Lim HK, Choi D, Lee WJ, et al. Hepatocellular carcinoma treated with percutaneous radiofrequency ablation: evaluation with follow-up multiphase helical CT. Radiology. 2001;221:447–54.
8. Dromain C, de Baere T, Elias D, et al. Hepatic tumors treated with percutaneous radio-frequency ablation: CT and MR imaging follow-up. Radiology. 2002;223:255–62.
9. Park Y, Choi D, Rhim H, et al. Central lower attenuating lesion in the ablation zone on immediate follow-up CT after percutaneous radiofrequency ablation for hepatocellular carcinoma: incidence and clinical significance. Eur J Radiol. 2010;75:391–6.
10. Kierans AS, Elazzazi M, Braga L, et al. Thermoablative treatments for malignant liver lesions: 10-year experience of MRI appearances of treatment response. AJR Am J Roentgenol. 2010;194:523–9.
11. Sainani NI, Gervais DA, Mueller PR, et al. Imaging after percutaneous radiofrequency ablation of hepatic tumors: part 2, abnormal findings. AJR Am J Roentgenol. 2013;200:194–204.
12. Shah PA, Cunningham SC, Morgan TA, et al. Hepatic gas: widening spectrum of causes detected at CT and US in the interventional era. Radiographics. 2011;31:1403–13.
13. Kim KW, Lee JM, Klotz E, et al. Safety margin assessment after radiofrequency ablation of the liver using registration of preprocedure and post-procedure CT images. AJR Am J Roentgenol. 2011; 196:W565–72.
14. Purandare NC, Rangarajan V, Shah SA, et al. Therapeutic response to radiofrequency ablation of neoplastic lesions: FDG PET/CT findings. Radiographics. 2011;31:201–13.
15. Goto E, Tateishi R, Shiina S, et al. Hemorrhagic complications of percutaneous radiofrequency ablation for liver tumors. J Clin Gastroenterol. 2010;44:374–80.
16. Chang IS, Rhim H, Kim SH, et al. Biloma formation after radiofrequency ablation of hepatocellular carcinoma: incidence, imaging features, and clinical significance. AJR Am J Roentgenol. 2010;195:1131–6.
17. Choi D, Lim HK, Kim MJ, et al. Liver abscess after percutaneous radiofrequency ablation for hepatocellular carcinomas: frequency and risk factors. AJR Am J Roentgenol. 2005;184:1860–7.
18. Ogawa T, Kawamoto H, Kobayashi Y, et al. Prevention of biliary complication in radiofrequency ablation for hepatocellular carcinoma-Cooling effect by endoscopic nasobiliary drainage tube. Eur J Radiol. 2010;73:385–90.
19. Maeda T, Hong J, Konishi K, et al. Tumor ablation therapy of liver cancers with an open magnetic resonance imaging-based navigation system. Surg Endosc. 2009;23:1048–53.
20. Yu H, Jang HJ, Kim TK, et al. Pseudoenhancement within the local ablation zone of hepatic tumors due to a nonlinear artifact on contrast-enhanced ultrasound. AJR Am J Roentgenol. 2010;194:653–9.
21. Sparchez Z, Radu P, Anton O, et al. Contrast enhanced ultrasound in assessing therapeutic response in ablative treatments of hepatocellular carcinoma. J Gastrointestin Liver Dis. 2009;18:243–8.
22. Eisele RM, Schumacher G, Lopez-Hänninen E, et al. Role of B-mode ultrasound screening in detection of local tumor recurrence in the first year after radiofrequency ablation in the liver. Cancer Detect Prev. 2007;31:316–22.
23. Harvey CJ, Blomley MJ, Eckersley RJ, et al. Hepatic malignancies: improved detection with pulse-inversion US in late phase of enhancement with SH U 508A-early experience. Radiology. 2000;216:903–8.
24. Leen E, Averkiou M, Arditi M, et al. Dynamic contrast enhanced ultrasound assessment of the vascular effects of novel therapeutics in early stage trials. Eur Radiol. 2012;22:1442–50.
25. Bargellini I, Bozzi E, Campani D, et al. Modified RECIST to assess tumor response after transarterial chemoembolization of hepatocellular carcinoma: CT-pathologic correlation in 178 liver explants. Eur J Radiol. 2013;82:e212–8.

# Adjuvant Therapy After Radiofrequency Ablation

# 10

Hengjun Gao and Minshan Chen

## 10.1 Introduction

It is commonly recognized that hepatocellular carcinoma (HCC) accounts for approximately 60–80 % recurrence rate after 5 years of radiofrequency thermal ablation (RFA) operation, even in small HCC patients who experienced complete ablative operation [1, 2]. Generally, HCC is considered to recur more frequently from intrahepatic remnant micrometastasis within 1–2 years after RFA (defined as "early recurrence"). The late recurrence (2 or more than 2 years) mainly ascribes to the carcinogenic effect of underlying chronic liver disease [3]. Regardless of early or late recurrence, the prevention of tumor recurrence is extremely important, but unmet clinical administration. Except for improving the ablative effect with update techniques, adjuvant therapy after RFA may probably prevent the recurrence and improve the overall survival curve in small HCC patients. Moreover, treatments to prevent tumor recurrence should be conducted in accordance with the potential mechanisms of recurrence. Several clinical strategies including antiviral therapy with interferon and nucleoside analogues, immunotherapy, biotherapy, etc., have been recommended as the therapeutic options for the prevention of tumor recurrence after RFA.

H. Gao, MD, PhD • M. Chen, MD, PhD (✉)
Department of Hepatobiliary Surgery, Sun Yat-sen University Cancer Center, Guangzhou, China
e-mail: chminsh@mail.sysu.edu.cn

## 10.2 Antiviral Therapy After RFA

In general, the main risk factor of HCC development is chronic infection with HBV and HCV. The high replication of hepatitis virus is associated with late recurrence of HCC. A correlation between higher serum virus load and increased risk of HCC recurrence after surgical resection has been confirmed [4]. Therefore, antiviral therapy to suppress the replication of hepatitis virus can theoretically reduce the recurrence rate and improve survival rate of HCC after RFA. Currently, many antiviral agents for the treatment of chronic hepatitis B infection are developed including interferon-α (IFN-α); nucleotide analogues (NAs) which include lamivudine, entecavir, tenofovir, and adefovir; etc. Meanwhile, interferon therapy is mainly used for treatment of chronic hepatitis C infection, which is able to inhibit virus replication and recover the liver functions.

NAs are molecules that act like nucleosides in DNA or RNA replication. They include a range of antiviral products used to inhibit virus replication in infected cells. The direct antitumor activity of NAs has not been reported. Lamivudine is a potent nucleoside analog reverse transcriptase inhibitor (nRTI) but shows no inhibitory effects on integrated HBV DNA. Thus, it does not possess the suppressive effect on de novo carcinogenesis since the HBV gene has been integrated into the host genome [5]. Considering the rela-

© Springer Science+Business Media Dordrecht 2016
M. Chen et al. (eds.), *Radiofrequency Ablation for Small Hepatocellular Carcinoma*,
DOI 10.1007/978-94-017-7258-7_10

tionship between HBV DNA level and HCC recurrence rate, NAs are applied for the prevention of HCC recurrence on the basis of their inhibitory effects to HBV DNA load, rather than their direct antitumor effects. Consequently, it avoids hepatocyte injury and abnormal regeneration, eventually reducing the genetic instability and HCC recurrence rates. Recently, Wu et al. reported [6] a nationwide cohort study in Taiwan, China, for investing the association between nucleoside analogue and risk of tumor recurrence in HCC patients with hepatitis B virus (HBV) infection after curative surgery. The tumor recurrence status between patients with ($n=4051$) or without ($n=518$) NAs was compared. The result indicated that the patients with NAs had a significantly lower 6-year HCC recurrence rate. On modified Cox regression analysis, in the group of patients with NAs, it was independently associated with a reduced risk of HCC recurrence. They concluded that the application of NAs provided a lower risk of HCC recurrence to patients with HBV-related HCC after liver resection. Chuma et al. also reported that the tumor recurrence rate was significantly decreased in patients receiving lamivudine before HCC occurred [7]. In a retrospective study [8], authors investigated the cumulative recurrence rates of HCC in 49 patients who underwent curative therapy for HBV-related HCC (liver resection, $n=31$; RFA, $n=18$), 16 patients among them received lamivudine and 33 patients did not. Although there was no significant difference of HCC recurrence rates found, hepatic function preservation and survival rate were improved in patients receiving lamivudine, which allowed the patients ease to accept the repeated curative operation if required. In addition, HBV reactivation after curative operation cannot be ignored although the incidence was relatively lower after RFA when compared with hepatic resection. HBV reactivation was a serious problem and may result in severe liver damage, even death. A retrospective study showed that in 33 HCC patients who received antiviral agents after RFA, the incidence of HBV reactivation was 0 % (0/33), while in patient without receiving antiviral treatment, the incidence was 7.6 % (7/92) [9]. Therefore, the antiviral therapy should

be recommended for patients who experienced RFA for HBV-related HCC treatment. At present, lamivudine, adefovir, and entecavir are commonly selected for NA therapy. Entecavir is reported to be more effective for rapid reduction of viral load compared with other agents and is a safe and well-tolerated agent for long-term treatment [10]. Furthermore, entecavir has a higher genetic barrier to the resistance mutation for itself.

In contrast to nucleoside analogs, interferon (IFN) therapy is able to enhance host immune responses and promote cellular immune responses to inhibit hepatitis virus replication and gene expression. IFN-α is an approved and effective agent for CHB treatment contributing to HBeAg seroconversion and histological remission in about one third of the patients. In addition, several studies suggested previously that IFN-α therapy might have long-term beneficial effects in terms of viral clearance, HCC prevention, and survival extension in patients with CHB [11]. Compared to nucleoside/nucleotide analogues, the advantages of IFN-α therapy included a more sustained virus response and lower drug-related resistance mutation. In HCV-infected patients, IFN is the first-line treatment to decrease the elevated serum alanine aminotransferase (ALT) levels and improve hepatic necroinflammation and fibrosis and then further remove the serum HCV-RNA in chronic hepatitis C patients. Besides, many experiments and clinical trials have shown that IFN is of antitumor effects and is capable of inhibiting the proliferation of cancer cells. Three possible mechanisms may be involved in anticancer effects. First, IFN induces cyclin-dependent kinase (CDK) inhibitors which affect G1/G0 arrest [12]. Second, IFN augments T-cell cytotoxicity and induces apoptosis of cancer cells via the immune system [13]. Thirdly, IFN inhibits tumor angiogenesis [14]. Therefore, we considered that IFN therapy could prevent the HCC recurrence after curative operation through the improvement of active hepatitis activity and hepatic fibrosis and the anticancer efficacy (Fig. 10.1).

In a retrospective study, Someya et al. [15] investigated the role of IFN in HCC patients with

**Fig. 10.1** Diagram of potential mechanisms of direct effect of IFN to antitumor growth

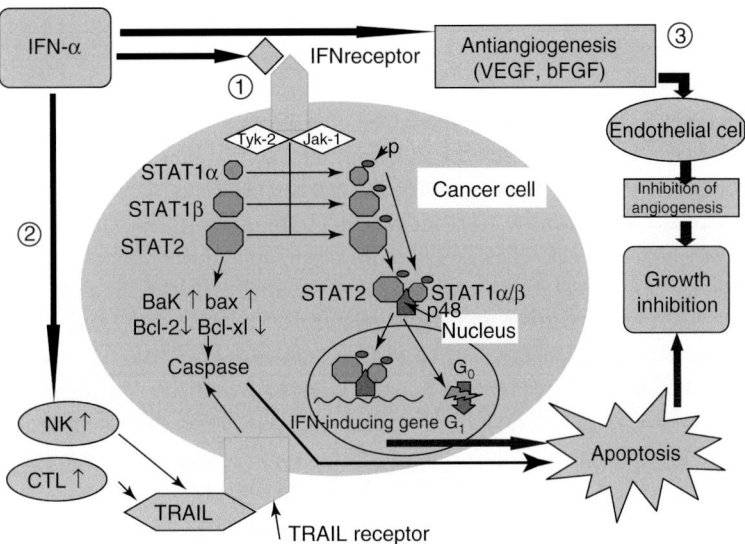

HBV-related cirrhosis after curative operation; the results showed that IFN prevented tumor recurrence, especially in those with higher aspartate transaminase levels. Furthermore, the randomized controlled trials (RCTs) have been conducted to explore the effects of IFN for preventing recurrences in HCC patients after treatment. Lo et al. [16] conducted an RCT in a series of 40 patients with HBV-related HCC after hepatic resection. Patients treated with IFN-α2b, 10 MU/m$^2$, three times a week for 12 weeks were compared with controls. The survival rates in the IFN-treated patients at 1st and 5th years after surgery were 97 % and 79 %, respectively, compared to 85 % and 61 % in the control. Multivariate analysis showed that IFN might decrease the risk of patient death. In a subgroup analysis, the 5-year survival rate in stage I/II patients did not show the difference between the IFN group and controls. However, the early recurrence rate in stage III/IVA HCC patients with IFN administered was significantly decreased, and the 5-year survival rate was improved from 24 to 68 %. Sun et al. [17] also demonstrated that postoperative IFN-α treatment postponed tumor recurrence and improved overall survival in HBV-related HCC patients after curative resection in an RCT study. Therefore, the therapeutic approach with IFN to prevent HCC recurrence after operation has been gradually adopted in clinical practice. Moreover,

conventional IFNs have been replaced gradually by a new pegylated (PEG)-IFN as a common agent due to its advantages of higher response rate and simpler management method, which needs to be taken once a week only, rather than daily or three times a week.

Nevertheless, of the case–control studies reported previously, five cases were associated to hepatitis C [18–20] and two cases were associated to hepatitis B-related HCC [15, 21]. Suou et al. [18] assessed whether IFN-α could inhibit intrahepatic recurrence in small HCC patients with underlying disease of chronic hepatitis C after curative operation. The data from 40 patients who were with solitary, small HCC (lesion ≤3 cm in diameter), underlying chronic hepatitis C, and age ≤70 years were analyzed. Among them, 18 patients were treated with IFN-α for 6 months after HCC operation and 22 patients without IFN-α therapy were used as controls. In which, six patients (33 %) in the IFN group showed sustained response, but the incidence of local recurrence did not show the significant difference (6 % vs. 9 %, $P > 0.05$). The cumulative incidences of distant recurrence in controls vs. the IFN group were 9 % and 6 % at year 1, 27 % and 11 % at year 2, 63 % and 18 % at year 3, 76 % and 28 % at year 4, and 82 % and 28 % at year 5, respectively, with a significant difference between the two groups. Six patients (27 %) in the non-IFN-treated group were dead with the progress of HCC, but all patients in the IFN-treated group were alive ($P$ <0.05). The pilot study demonstrated that IFN-α therapy for small HCC patients after curative operation could inhibit intrahepatic recurrence in the residual liver and improved prognosis of hepatitis C virus-related HCC. Hung et al. [20] reported that antiviral therapy suppressed tumor recurrence and influenced overall survival rate in patients with HCV-related HCC, who had complete ablation of nodules by nonsurgical treatments. Twenty HCC patients with three or less HCV-related nodules were treated with percutaneous tumor ablation and/or transcatheter arterial embolization combined with interferon (IFN; 3 or 5 million units of IFN alpha-2b thrice a week) plus ribavirin (1000–1200 mg per day) for 24–48 weeks after complete ablation of lesions. During the same period, additional 40 age- and sex-matched patients with similar characteristics of tumors (sizes, numbers, and treatment modalities) and severity of liver disease were recruited as controls. In 20 patients with antiviral therapy, 16 completed therapy and 10 showed a sustained response with normalization of alanine aminotransferase and negative HCV-RNA at 6 months after therapy completion. Since treated child B patients experienced severe side effects (most patients then discontinued antiviral therapy), clinical outcomes were analyzed only in the treated child A patients ($n$ = 16) vs. controls ($n$ = 33). There was no significant difference in the local recurrence incidence in patients with sustained response compared to those without response or subjects as controls. However, the second recurrence-free interval and survival in patients with sustained response was significantly longer than those in patients without response and subjects in controls. These results indicated that successful antiviral therapy for HCV-related HCC patients after nonsurgical tumor ablation may lower tumor recurrence rate and prolong the survival. Qu et al. [21] retrospectively analyzed the effect of IFN-α therapy on survival and tumor recurrence in patients with HBV-related HCC after curative resection. A total of 568 HBV-related HCC patients had undergone curative resection. Among them, 101 patients received

postoperative IFN-α therapy (5 million units, 3 times a week for 18 months) with median follow-up of 53.3 months. The results indicated that patients with postoperative IFN-α therapy showed higher overall survival rates, whereas no significant difference was found in disease-free survival rates between the two groups. Multivariate analysis revealed that postoperative IFN-α therapy was an independent factor for overall survival and could significantly reduce the risk of early tumor recurrence. Therefore, IFN-α given after curative resection could inhibit the early tumor reappearance and improve the overall survival in patients with HBV-related HCC.

The tumor recurrence and survival rate were evaluated similarly in all of these RCT studies. Significant differences were shown of the survival rate in subjects with a prolonged IFN administration. Improvements of survival rate were observed in one study with 6-month administration [18, 20] and another study with a median administration of 4.7 years [22]. A significant difference of tumor recurrence rate (including the rates of the second and third recurrences) was noted in all three studies. It was also reported recently that the tumor recurrence was significantly suppressed, and the survival was prolonged in patients administered with IFN for 2 years or longer [23]. Also, the recurrence rate of HBV-related HCC and the hazard ratio were lowered in IFN-treated patients than those in patients without IFN treatment [15]. IFN administration has also been reported to increase the overall survival rate [21]. These results suggested that the effect of IFN for preventing the tumor recurrence might be through the mechanisms of suppressing the inflammation or direct anticancer effect to both hepatitis C and B patients.

In addition, IFN has been proposed [19, 22] to be used at a low dosage for longer term consecutively as a maintenance therapy to improve the ALT level and expect its direct anticancer effect, rather than to eliminate the virus. In a report about IFN maintenance therapy, a total of 127 HCC patients (tumor diameter ≤3 cm; number of tumors ≤3) were performed RFA curatively. Among them, 43 patients received 3,000,000 IU

IFN-α2b twice per week or PEG IFN-α2a 90 μg once per week or once per 2 weeks without discontinuation (IFN group maintenance). Meanwhile, additional 84 patients did not receive IFN treatment (control group). The data showed that the 5-year survival rate was 66 % in the control group and 83 % in the IFN group maintenance ($p=0.004$). Multivariate analysis using the Cox proportional hazards model identified IFN maintenance therapy as an independent risk factor for survival, and the risk ratio was 0.21 (95 % CI: 0.05–0.73). Therefore, the authors concluded that the curative protocol of IFN at low dose for long-term maintenance after RFA operation significantly delayed the first recurrence, prevent the second and third recurrences, and consequently improved survival (Table 10.1) [22, 24].

According to Jeong et al. [25], the Child–Pugh score did not show the difference in IFN-treated patients, but was significantly deteriorated in controls during the follow-up period. The percentage of patients who were unable to be a candidate for surgery due to extensive cancerometastasis or worsening liver function was increased in the control group than those in the IFN group. In summary, the regimen of IFN therapy with long-term maintenance at low dosage seemed able to significantly prevent or delay the recurrence of HCC and the occurring of secondary carcinogenesis by preserving the liver function in an adequate state or by its direct anticancer effect, which made it possible to detect a slight recurrence and improve the survival rate while disease was still staying in a relatively early stage and the curative operation was allowed again. In addition, the performance of noncurative treatments such as transarterial chemoembolization which would damage the liver function and IFN therapy which might preserve the liver function was required to be considered meticulously for improving the survival rate [24].

## 10.3 Immunotherapy After RFA

RFA-induced high temperature caused coagulation necrosis of HCC mass, which collapsed body's immune suppression status by reducing the tumor burden, increased the exposure of tumor cell epitopes and promoted the synthesis of heat shock protein (HSP), thereby effectively activated the antitumor immune response. The cytokine and/or chemokine milieu might also enhance the antineoplastic function and stimulated the recruitment of circulating immune cells to tumor site. Moreover, many studies proposed that RFA could act as a strong "adjuvant" for antitumor responses and induce antigen-presenting cell infiltration and the amplification of weak tumor-induced immunity. RFA could

**Table 10.1** Therapeutic effect of interferon to patients with hepatocellular carcinoma (HCC) after surgical procedure

| Study | With vs. without INF ($n$) | Etiology | Follow-up | HCC treatment modality | P value (recurrence) | P value (survival) |
|---|---|---|---|---|---|---|
| Someya et al. | 11 vs. 69 | HBV | 3 years | Ablation | NS ($P=0.0139$) | NA |
| Lo et al. | 40 vs. 40 | HBV/HCV | 5 years | Resection | $P<0.05$ (early recurrence) | $P=0.038$ (stage III/IVA) |
| Sun et al. | 118 vs. 118 | HBV | 36.6 months (median) | Resection | $P<0.048$ | $P<0.0003$ |
| Suou et al. | 18 vs. 22 | HCV | 5 years | Resection/RFA | $P<0.01$ | $P<0.05$ |
| Sakaguchi et al. | 24 vs. 33 | HCV | 3 years | RFA | $P<0.02$ | NS |
| Hung et al. | 20 vs. 40 | HCV | 6 months | RFA/TACE | $P=0.0141$ | NS |
| Qu et al. | 101 vs. 467 | HBV | 53.3 months (median) | Resection | $P=0.005$ (early recurrence) | $P=0.01$ |
| Kudo et al. | 43 vs. 84 | HCV | 5 years | RFA | $P<0.05$ | 0.004 |
| Ikeda et al. | 77 vs. 302 | HCV | 5 years | RFA | $P<0.05$ | NA |

Note: *NS* not significant, *NA* not available

also induce a tumor-specific proliferative T-cell response, even transplantable protective immunity, but not activating the increase of CD4+CD25+Foxp3+ regulatory T cells compared those in patients treated with surgical resection. However, this RFA alone-stimulated tumor-specific immune response did not appear to be sufficient enough to control HCC. It provided the strategy for the development of a potential adjuvant immunotherapy in patients undergoing RFA. So far, a series of pilot studies have showed inspiring data, and the authors proposed that adoptive immunotherapy after RFA was a safe and effective therapeutic modality for HCC patients. Weng et al. [26] reported the administration of cytokine-induced killer (CIK) cell immunotherapy was helpful in the clearance of microscopic residual tumors and the prevention of recurrence after TACE and RFA management in HCC patients. In this study, 85 HCC patients after transcatheter arterial chemoembolization (TACE) and RFA therapy were randomized to group with immunotherapy and group without adjuvant therapy. Autologous cytokine-induced killer (CIK) cells were transfused via hepatic artery to the patients. Interestingly, with the infusion of CIK cells, the percentages of CD3+, CD4+, CD56+, and CD3+CD56+ cells and CD4+/CD8+ ratio were significantly increased compared with the baseline, respectively, whereas the percentage of CD8+ cells was decreased from $31.1 \pm 7.8$ to $28.6 \pm 8.3$ %. The recurrence rates at 12 months and 18 months in the treated group were 8.9 % and 15.6 %, respectively, compared with 30.0 % and 40.0 % in controls. These outcomes suggested that transfusion of CIK cells was a feasible and effective treatment. It could boost the immunologic functions in HCC patients and play an important role in reducing the recurrence rate of HCC. The possible mechanism may involve the property of CIK cells migrating toward the tumor sites and play an antitumor activity. CIK cells are also used as carriers for virus to induce tumor cell lysis. The cytotoxicity to tumor cells is non-major histocompatibility complex restricted, relies on cell–cell contact, and is perforin dependent and eFas independent. The higher lytic activity of CIK cells is mainly due to the higher

proliferation of CD3 and CD56 double positive cells. Another feature of CIK cells is the production of effector cytokines such as IFN-γ and a number of chemokines including RANTES, MIP-1α, and MIP-1β. These chemokines function together with IFN-γ, enabling them to potentially tilt the immune response toward a Th1 direction.

Another report [27] investigated the effects of combination of RFA with autologous RetroNectin-activated killer (RAK) cells in the treatment of small HCC. RetroNectin is a recombinant human fibronectin fragment (CH-296) for increasing retroviral-mediated gene transduction by colocalizing target cells and virions on the rFN-CH296 molecules. In the present study, stimulated by immobilized RetroNectin and anti-CD3mAb, a high yield of RAK cells was obtained at a range of $1.17 \times 10^{10} - 2.58 \times 10^{10}$ cells on each harvest and a distinguishable population of CD3+CD8+ and CD45RA+ cells. RFA was first used to lower the tumor burdens in HCC patients, followed by six sessions of RAK cell infusions. After combination treatment, CD3+CD8+ and IFN-γ were increased significantly in patients' peripheral blood. After the 7-month follow-up, no severe adverse events, tumor recurrences, and death case were observed in the total of seven HCC patients, indicating the safety and efficacy of the combination of RFA and RAK cell adoptive immunotherapy in HCC treatment.

In addition, RFA operation increased circulating pool of NK lymphocytes in peripheral blood in HCC patients. The effect of RFA did not appear simply limited to peripheral mobilization because relevant aspects of the NK population, including the subset composition, expression of activatory and inhibitory receptors, direct and indirect IgG-mediated cytotoxicity, and potential for IFN-γ secretion, were also significantly and consistently increased. Interestingly, all NK modifications were oriented toward a more differentiated and proactivatory phenotype with a general increase of functional activities typical of cytotoxic/effector cells. These correlates corroborate hypothesis that the overall effect on the NK-cell pool could make part of RFA-driven anticancer immune stimulation in liver cancer patients. The increase of circulating NK cells was not so impressive in quantitative term; however, the general effect was consistent and persistent in the entire observation period with significant difference statically. Moreover, the increase of peripheral NK-cell pool is not attributable to tumor burden relief but to the stimulation of RFA. Based on the acknowledgement of multiple mechanisms of RFA-stimulated immunological effect, Cui et al. [28] reported a pilot study involving cellular immunotherapy (CIT) adopting multiple types of cells combined with RFA for HCC patients' treatment. 62 HCC patients treated with radical RFA were divided into two groups: RFA alone ($n = 32$) and RFA/CIT ($n = 30$). Autologous mononuclear cells were collected and then induced into natural killer (NK) cells, $\gamma\delta$ T cells, and cytokine-induced killer (CIK) cells. These cells were identified by flow cytometry with their specific antibodies and were infused intravenously to RFA/CIT patients for three or six sessions thereafter. The results implied that progression-free survival (PFS) was higher in the RFA/CIT group than that in the RFA group. In the RFA/CIT group, six sessions of infusion demonstrated a better survival curve than three courses of infusion. Viral load of hepatitis C was decreased in two of three patients without antiviral therapy in the RFA/CIT group but was increased in the RFA group. No significant adverse events were found in the patients with CIT. The novel study indicated that combination of sequential CIT with RFA for HCC patients was efficient and safe and may be helpful in the prevention of recurrence for the patients with HCC after RFA.

Another mechanism that modulates tumor-specific T-cell response after RFA in HCC patients is that RFA can provide the appropriate stimuli for maturation of both immature monocyte-derived dendritic cells (MoDCs) and monocytes activated by granulocyte macrophage colony-stimulating factor (GM-CSF). Tumor debris lysates of thermally ablated HCC nodules promoted upregulation of costimulatory molecules, improved the antigen-presenting function of DCs, and eventually triggered an efficient tumor-specific T-cell response. Based on these explanations, exploiting the "adjuvant" effect of RFA to allow final differentiation of intralesionally injected APCs and presentation of tumor antigens in an optimal immunostimulatory milieu for triggering effector antitumor T-cell responses finically play a role in the clearance of remnant tumor cell. By basic experiments, Liu et al. [29] investigated a prime-boost strategy combining a prime with heat-shocked tumor cell lysate-pulsed dendritic cell (HT-DC) followed by an in situ boost with RFA. The combination treatment with HT-DC and RFA showed potent antitumor effects, with $\geq 90$ % of tumor recurrence abrogated following RFA treatment. By contrast, pre-vaccination with unheated tumor lysate-pulsed DC had little effect on tumor relapse. Analysis of the underlying mechanism revealed that spleno-cytes from mice treated with HT-DC plus RFA contained significantly more tumor-specific, IFN-$\gamma$-secreting T cells compared with control groups. Moreover, adoptive transfer of spleno-cytes from successfully treated tumor-free mice protected naive animals from tumor recurrence following RFA, and this was mediated mainly by CD8+ T cells. Therefore, the optimal priming for the DC vaccination before RFA is important for boosting antigen-specific T-cell responses and prevention of cancer recurrence.

Besides, RFA-combined interleukin-2 (IL-2) therapy induced the highest levels of macrophage recruitment and dendritic cell migration resulting in enhanced CTL activity, increased tumor apoptosis, elevated systemic antitumor immunity, and the best inhibition of tumor growth. IL-2 is a major regulator of the immune system and an important element to stimulate the immune system for fighting cancer. IL-2 acts as a growth factor for T lymphocytes and also as a promoter for the activities of monocytes/macrophages, natural killer cells (NK cells), and neutrophils. Activated cytotoxic cells induce apoptosis and kill tumor cells through a perforin-granzyme-mediated signaling or a Fas-mediated pathway. Some preliminary studies have demonstrated certain success in tumor regression through administration of IL-2 systemically. However, IL-2 treatment induced severe side effects when administered systemically and its half-life was only $2.9 \pm 0.5$ min after

IV injection. Local delivery of cytokines was expected to overcome these disadvantages, and several clinical trials have been performed to verify the outcome. Results included regression of tumor size in 25 % of the patients, extension of disease-free survival period, and activation of immune cells including T cells, NK cells, CD25[+] cells, and HLA DR[+] cells. Recently, a gene delivery system was developed with promising antitumor effects. Suppression of tumor growth, enhanced CTL, NK-cell activity, prevention of NKG2D suppression, induction of tumor cell apoptosis, and synergistic antitumor activity occurred when IL-2 gene therapy was combined with local herpes thymidine kinase gene delivery, systemic administration of cisplatin, or external-beam radiation therapy. Therefore, additional IL-2 gene therapy is expected to possess a high potential to enhance the antitumoral immune response induced by RFA [30].

# References

1. Huang J, Yan L, Cheng Z, et al. A randomized trial comparing radiofrequency ablation and surgical resection for HCC conforming to the Milan criteria. Ann Surg. 2010;252:903–12.
2. Lencioni R, Cioni D, Crocetti L, et al. Early-stage hepatocellular carcinoma in patients with cirrhosis: long-term results of percutaneous image-guided radiofrequency ablation. Radiology. 2005;234:961–7.
3. Imamura H, Matsuyama Y, Tanaka E, et al. Risk factors contributing to early and late phase intrahepatic recurrence of hepatocellular carcinoma after hepatectomy. J Hepatol. 2003;38:200–7.
4. Kim BK, Park JY, Kim dY, et al. Persistent hepatitis B viral replication affects recurrence of hepatocellular carcinoma after curative resection. Liver Int. 2008;28:393–401.
5. Matsumoto A, Tanaka E, Rokuhara A, et al. Efficacy of lamivudine for preventing hepatocellular carcinoma in chronic hepatitis B: A multicenter retrospective study of 2795 patients. Hepatol Res. 2005;32:173–84.
6. Wu CY, Chen YJ, Ho HJ, et al. Association between nucleoside analogues and risk of hepatitis B virus–related hepatocellular carcinoma recurrence following liver resection. JAMA. 2012;308:1906–14.
7. Chuma M, Hige S, Kamiyama T, et al. The influence of hepatitis B DNA level and antiviral therapy on recurrence after initial curative treatment in patients

with hepatocellular carcinoma. J Gastroenterol. 2009;44:991–9.
8. Kuzuya T, Katano Y, Kumada T, et al. Efficacy of antiviral therapy with lamivudine after initial treatment for hepatitis B virus-related hepatocellular carcinoma. J Gastroenterol Hepatol. 2007;22:1929–35.
9. Dan JQ, Zhang YJ, Huang JT, et al. Hepatitis B virus reactivation after radiofrequency ablation or hepatic resection for HBV-related small hepatocellular carcinoma: a retrospective study. Eur J Surg Oncol. 2013;39:865–72.
10. Chang TT, Gish RG, de Man R, et al. A comparison of entecavir and lamivudine for HBeAg-positive chronic hepatitis B. N Engl J Med. 2006;354:1001–10.
11. Senturk H, Baysal B, Tahan V, et al. Long-term effect of interferon therapy in patients with HBeAg positive chronic hepatitis B infection. Dig Dis Sci. 2011;56:208–12.
12. Takaoka A, Hayakawa S, Yanai H, et al. Integration of interferon-alpha/beta signalling to p53 responses in tumour suppression and antiviral defence. Nature. 2003;424:516–23.
13. Lindahl P, Leary P, Gresser I. Enhancement by interferon of the specific cytotoxicity of sensitized lymphocytes. Proc Natl Acad Sci U S A. 1972;69:721–5.
14. Folkman J, Ingber D. Inhibition of angiogenesis. Semin Cancer Biol. 1992;3:89–96.
15. Someya T, Ikeda K, Saitoh S, et al. Interferon lowers tumor recurrence rate after surgical resection or ablation of hepatocellular carcinoma: a pilot study of patients with hepatitis B virus-related cirrhosis. J Gastroenterol. 2006;41:1206–13.
16. Lo CM, Liu CL, Chan SC, et al. A randomized, controlled trial of postoperative adjuvant interferon therapy after resection of hepatocellular carcinoma. Ann Surg. 2007;245:831–42.
17. Sun HC, Tang ZY, Wang L, et al. Postoperative interferon alpha treatment postponed recurrence and improved overall survival in patients after curative resection of HBV-related hepatocellular carcinoma: a randomized clinical trial. J Cancer Res Clin Oncol. 2006;132:458–65.
18. Suou T, Mitsuda A, Koda M, et al. Interferon alpha inhibits intrahepatic recurrence in hepatocellular carcinoma with chronic hepatitis C: a pilot study. Hepatol Res. 2001;20:301–11.
19. Sakaguchi Y, Kudo M, Fukunaga T, et al. Low-dose, long-term, intermittent interferon-alpha-2b therapy after radical treatment by radiofrequency ablation delays clinical recurrence in patients with hepatitis C virus-related hepatocellular carcinoma. Intervirology. 2005;48:64–70.
20. Hung CH, Lee CM, Wang JH, et al. Antiviral therapy after non-surgical tumor ablation in patients with hepatocellular carcinoma associated with hepatitis C virus. J Gastroenterol Hepatol. 2005;20:1553–9.
21. Qu LS, Jin F, Huang XW, et al. Interferon-α therapy after curative resection prevents early recurrence and improves survival in patients with hepatitis B virus-

related hepatocellular carcinoma. J Surg Oncol. 2010;102:796–801.

22. Kudo M, Sakaguchi Y, Chung H, et al. Long-term interferon maintenance therapy improves survival in patients with HCV-related hepatocellular carcinoma after curative radiofrequency ablation. A matched case–control study. Oncology. 2007;72 Suppl 1:132–8.

23. Ikeda K, Kobayashi M, Seko Y, et al. Administration of interferon for two or more years decreases early stage hepatocellular carcinoma recurrence rate after radical ablation: a retrospective study of hepatitis C virus-related liver cancer. Hepatol Res. 2010;40:1168–75.

24. Kudo M. Impact of interferon therapy after curative treatment of hepatocellular carcinoma. Oncology. 2008;75 Suppl 1:30–41.

25. Jeong S, Aikata H, Katamura Y, et al. Low-dose intermittent interferon-alpha therapy for HCV-related liver cirrhosis after curative treatment of hepatocellular carcinoma. World J Gastroenterol. 2007;13:5188–95.

26. Weng DS, Zhou J, Zhou QM, et al. Minimally invasive treatment combined with cytokine-induced killer cells therapy lower the short-term recurrence rates of hepatocellular carcinomas. J Immunother. 2008;31:63–71.

27. Ma H, Zhang Y, Wang Q, et al. Therapeutic safety and effects of adjuvant autologous RetroNectin activated killer cell immunotherapy for patients with primary hepatocellular carcinoma after radiofrequency ablation. Cancer Biol Ther. 2010;9:903–7.

28. Cui J, Wang N, Zhao H, et al. Combination of radiofrequency ablation and sequential cellular immunotherapy improves progression-free survival for patients with hepatocellular carcinoma. Int J Cancer. 2014;134:342–51.

29. Liu Q, Zhai B, Yang W, et al. Abrogation of local cancer recurrence after radiofrequency ablation by dendritic cell-based hyperthermic tumor vaccine. Mol Ther. 2009;17:2049–57.

30. Saito K, Araki K, Reddy N, et al. Enhanced local dendritic cell activity and tumor-specific immunoresponse in combined radiofrequency ablation and interleukin-2 for the treatment of human head and neck cancer in a murine orthotopic model. Head Neck. 2011;33:359–67.

# Surgery vs. Radiofrequency Ablation for Small Hepatocellular Carcinoma

# 11

Zoe Thompson, Tamara Gall, and Long R. Jiao

## 11.1 Introduction

Whilst the management of unresectable hepatocellular carcinoma (HCC) is well established, there remains great debate between interventional radiologists and hepatic surgeons as to the best treatment option for patients with small resectable HCC. Historically, where liver transplantation is not possible, treatment has been in the form of hepatic resection (HR). However, recent advances have seen an increasing use of local ablative therapies with laser and radiofrequency for management of resectable HCC. Radiofrequency ablation (RFA) is now being used more frequently, particularly when HCC is small. Interventional radiologists would argue that although surgical resection is a mainstay of treatment, it can compromise the function of already cirrhotic livers, in which case RFA may be a more appropriate form of treatment. However, hepatic surgeons would argue that RFA is not always able to achieve complete and sustained tumour necrosis coupled with evidence of micro metastases from tumour dissemination with local ablative therapy. For these reasons,

debate continues to exist regarding the most efficacious form of treatment.

In this chapter, we will review and analyse the currently available and published data to examine the effectiveness and efficacy of surgical resection and radiofrequency ablation in the treatment of hepatocellular carcinoma. We have conducted an extensive literature review by identifying all studies directly comparing hepatic resection with RFA for the treatment of hepatocellular carcinoma. Three randomised controlled trials (RCTs) were found, together with several other nonrandomised controlled trials [1–3].

## 11.2 Evidence

### 11.2.1 Randomised Control Trials and Meta-analysis

#### 11.2.1.1 Summary

There have been three randomised controlled trials (RCTs) comparing hepatectomy to radiofrequency ablation in HCC, published between 2006 and 2012 [1–3]. A recent meta-analysis combined these with several nonrandomised controlled trials (NRCTs) in order to increase the evidence base.

Chen et al. published the first study in 2006, involving 90 patients allocated to resection and 71 patients allocated to ablation [1]. Their results demonstrated a higher overall survival (73.4 % vs. 71.4 %) and disease-free survival (69.0 % vs.

Z. Thompson, MD, FRCS • T. Gall, MD, FRCS
L.R. Jiao, MD, FRCS (✉)
Department of Surgery and Cancer, Hammersmith Campus, Imperial College London, London, UK
e-mail: l.jiao@imperial.ac.uk

© Springer Science+Business Media Dordrecht 2016
M. Chen et al. (eds.), *Radiofrequency Ablation for Small Hepatocellular Carcinoma*,
DOI 10.1007/978-94-017-7258-7_11

64.1 %) at 3 years in the group allocated to resection compared to those undergoing ablation. These results were not statistically significant, and there was no difference when patients were stratified by tumour size. Ablation did demonstrate an advantage in less post-treatment complications, less pain and a shorter hospital admission.

Huang et al. published their study in 2010, with 115 patients allocated to resection and 115 to ablation [2]. Their 5-year survival rates were 75.7 % and 54.8 %, respectively ($p=0.001$). Their recurrence-free survival rates were 51.3 % for those in the resection group vs. 28.7 % for those undergoing ablation ($p=0.017$). The benefit of resection demonstrated was maintained when patients were stratified by tumour size and number.

The most recent RCT, published by Feng et al. in 2012, allocated 84 patients each to undergo resection or ablation [3]. Three-year survival rates were 74.8 % following surgery and 67.2 % following ablation ($p=0.342$), with corresponding recurrence-free survival quoted at 61.1 % and 49.6 %, respectively ($p=0.122$).

Of these three trials, only the study by Huang et al. demonstrated any statistical significance, with resection being favoured over ablation, in terms of both overall survival and recurrence-free survival. Their 5-year overall survival rate in the RFA group was significantly lower than HR ($p=0.001$) in tumours smaller than 5 cm.

In addition to the RCTs, the results from the nonrandomised controlled trials (NRCTs) were pooled in order to provide more information. This also demonstrated significantly lower overall survival rates in the RFA group, although the level of evidence was considerably lower.

## 11.2.1.2 Results of Intervention Based on Tumour Size

### Tumour Size ≤5 cm

#### Overall Survival

The meta-analysis of the three RCTs showed no significant difference between groups at 1 and 3 years. Huang et al. were the only group to look at survival at 5 years, which demonstrated a significantly better overall survival in the HR group ($p=0.001$).

Of the nonrandomised controlled trials, overall survival in the HR group was significantly better at 1 and 3 years, although the level of evidence was lower (Fig. 11.1).

#### Recurrence-Free Survival

Again, the RCTs showed no significant difference in recurrence-free survival rates at 1 and 3 years; however, the 5-year survival rate in the HR group was significantly better at 5 years.

The NRCTs demonstrated better survival rates at 1, 3 and 5 years in the HR group, although there was no significant difference between groups of 5-year recurrence-free survival rates for patients with Child-Pugh class A (Fig. 11.2).

#### Disease-Free Survival

The disease-free survival rate was only reported in one RCT, which demonstrated no difference between the two groups.

The pooled meta-analysis of the NRCTs showed significantly higher disease-free survival rates in the HR group at 1, 3 and 5 years.

#### Recurrence

The pooled results of the RCTs showed no significant difference at 1 year in recurrence rates (either local or distant), between the two groups. However, at 3 and 5 years, recurrence rates were significantly higher in the RFA group.

The meta-analysis of the NRCTs showed higher recurrence rates at 1, 3 and 5 years in the RFA group overall, although there were no significant differences between groups for patients with Child-Pugh Class A (Fig. 11.3).

#### In-Hospital Mortality, Complication Rate and Length of Hospital Stay

There were no significant differences in either the RCTs or the NRCTs regarding in-hospital mortality. The complication rate was lower in the RFA group, as evidenced by both RCTs and NRCTs. Length of hospital stay was 8.77 days shorter in the RCTs and 6.74 days fewer in the NRCTs (Fig. 11.4).

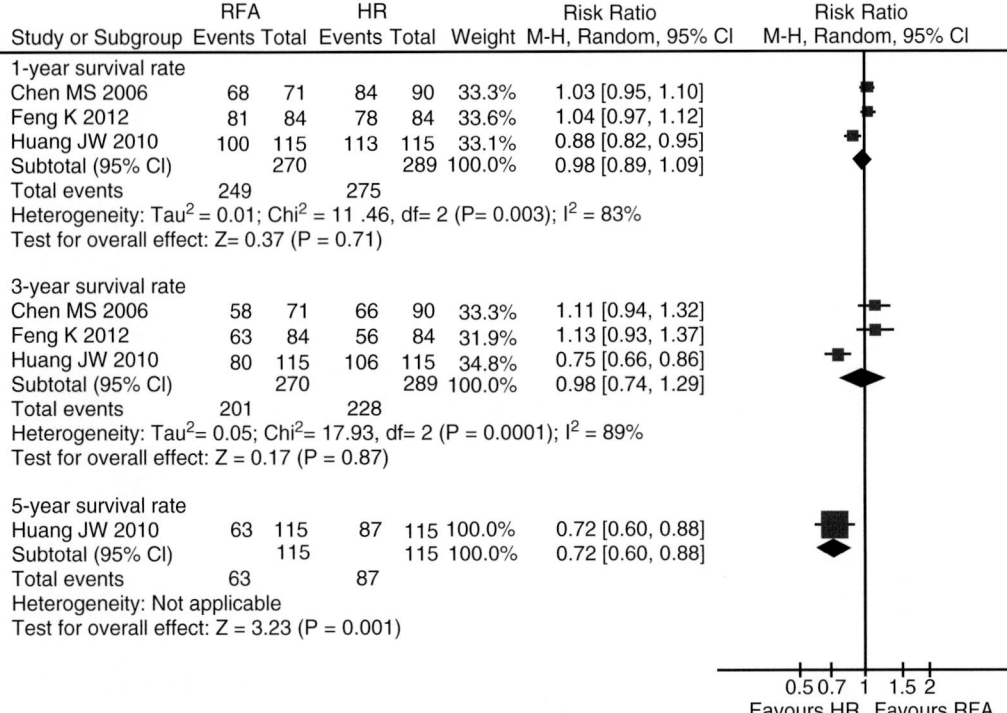

**Fig. 11.1** Overall survival (OS) at 1, 3 and 5 years in RCTs (Reprint from Yingqiang Wang et al. [5])

| Study or Subgroup | RFA Events | Total | HR Events | Total | Weight | Risk Ratio M-H, Random, 95% CI |
|---|---|---|---|---|---|---|
| **1-year survival rate** | | | | | | |
| Chen MS 2006 | 68 | 71 | 84 | 90 | 33.3% | 1.03 [0.95, 1.10] |
| Feng K 2012 | 81 | 84 | 78 | 84 | 33.6% | 1.04 [0.97, 1.12] |
| Huang JW 2010 | 100 | 115 | 113 | 115 | 33.1% | 0.88 [0.82, 0.95] |
| Subtotal (95% CI) | | 270 | | 289 | 100.0% | 0.98 [0.89, 1.09] |
| Total events | 249 | | 275 | | | |

Heterogeneity: Tau$^2$ = 0.01; Chi$^2$ = 11.46, df= 2 (P= 0.003); I$^2$ = 83%
Test for overall effect: Z= 0.37 (P = 0.71)

| | | | | | | |
|---|---|---|---|---|---|---|
| **3-year survival rate** | | | | | | |
| Chen MS 2006 | 58 | 71 | 66 | 90 | 33.3% | 1.11 [0.94, 1.32] |
| Feng K 2012 | 63 | 84 | 56 | 84 | 31.9% | 1.13 [0.93, 1.37] |
| Huang JW 2010 | 80 | 115 | 106 | 115 | 34.8% | 0.75 [0.66, 0.86] |
| Subtotal (95% CI) | | 270 | | 289 | 100.0% | 0.98 [0.74, 1.29] |
| Total events | 201 | | 228 | | | |

Heterogeneity: Tau$^2$= 0.05; Chi$^2$= 17.93, df= 2 (P = 0.0001); I$^2$ = 89%
Test for overall effect: Z = 0.17 (P = 0.87)

| | | | | | | |
|---|---|---|---|---|---|---|
| **5-year survival rate** | | | | | | |
| Huang JW 2010 | 63 | 115 | 87 | 115 | 100.0% | 0.72 [0.60, 0.88] |
| Subtotal (95% CI) | | 115 | | 115 | 100.0% | 0.72 [0.60, 0.88] |
| Total events | 63 | | 87 | | | |

Heterogeneity: Not applicable
Test for overall effect: Z = 3.23 (P = 0.001)

**Fig. 11.2** Recurrence-free survival rate (RFS) at 1, 3 and 5 years in RCTs (Reprint from Yingqiang Wang et al. [5])

| Study or Subgroup | RFA Events | Total | HR Events | Total | Weight | Risk Ratio M-H, Random, 95% CI |
|---|---|---|---|---|---|---|
| **1-year recurrence-free survival** | | | | | | |
| Feng K 2012 | 76 | 84 | 72 | 84 | 51.1% | 1.06 [0.94, 1.18] |
| Huang JW 2010 | 94 | 115 | 98 | 115 | 48.9% | 0.96 [0.85, 1.08] |
| Subtotal (95% CI) | | 199 | | 199 | 100.0% | 1.01 [0.92, 1.11] |
| Total events | 170 | | 170 | | | |

Heterogeneity: Tau$^2$ = 0.00; Chi$^2$= 1.41, df= 1 (P = 0.24); I$^2$= 29%
Test for overall effect: Z = 0.15 (P = 0.88)

| | | | | | | |
|---|---|---|---|---|---|---|
| **3-year recurrence-free survival** | | | | | | |
| Feng K 2012 | 51 | 84 | 42 | 84 | 49.1% | 1.21 [0.92, 1.60] |
| Huang JW 2010 | 53 | 115 | 70 | 115 | 50.9% | 0.76 [0.59, 0.97] |
| Subtotal (95% CI) | | 199 | | 199 | 100.0% | 0.95 (0.60, 1.52] |
| Total events | 104 | | 112 | | | |

Heterogeneity: Tau$^2$= 0.09; Chi$^2$= 6.31, df= 1 (P = 0.01); I$^2$= 84%
Test for overall effect: Z = 0.20 (P = 0.85)

| | | | | | | |
|---|---|---|---|---|---|---|
| **5-year recurrence-free survival** | | | | | | |
| Huang JW 2010 | 33 | 115 | 59 | 115 | 100.0% | 0.56 [0.40, 0.78] |
| Subtotal (95% CI) | | 115 | | 115 | 100.0% | 0.56 [0.40, 0.78] |
| Total events | 33 | | 59 | | | |

Heterogeneity: Not applicable
Test for overall effect: z = 3.36 (P = 0.0008)

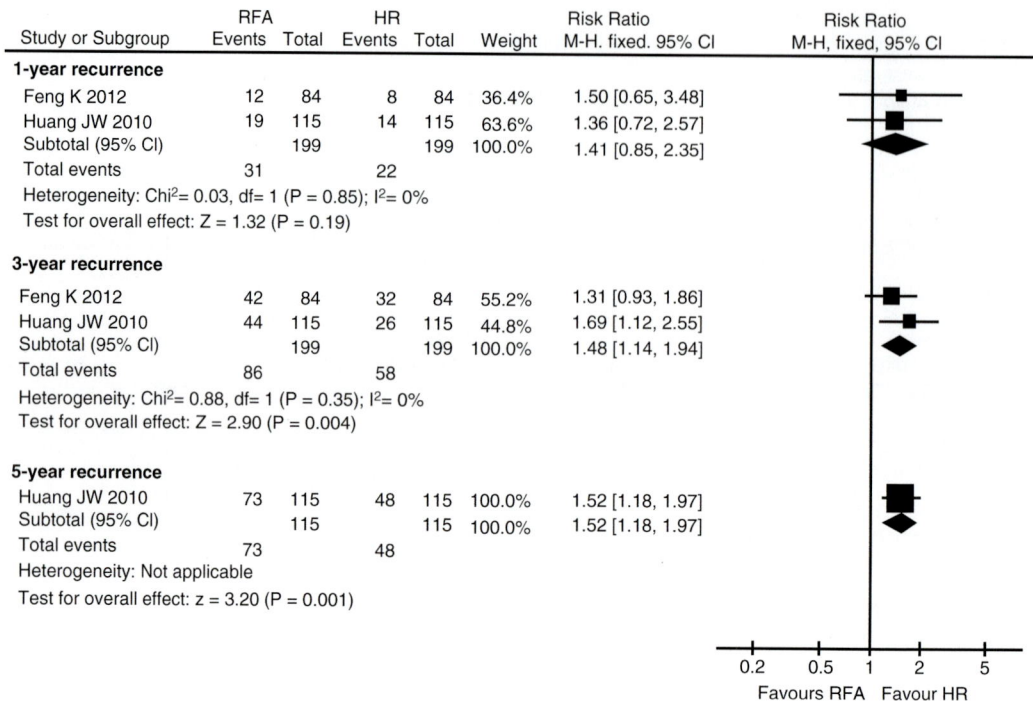

**Fig. 11.3** Recurrence rate at 1, 3 and 5 years in RCTs (Reprint from Yingqiang Wang et al. [5])

**Fig. 11.4** Complication rate of RCTs (Reprint from Yingqiang Wang et al. [5])

## Tumour Size 3–5 cm

Pooled results from the RCTs showed no significant difference of overall survival rates between the two groups for single HCC patients with this tumour size. NRCTs showed no difference at 1 and 3 years, although the 5-year survival rate in the HR group was higher. The 1, 3 and 5 year disease-free survival rates in the HR group were higher than the RFA group.

## Solitary Tumour <2 cm

Of the three RCTs, none specifically analysed the outcomes of these tumours; however, four

observational retrospective studies did so. None of these reported a convincing comparison between the two treatment arms, with the most frequent differences observed in RFA patients that were older, had a lower platelet count, more frequently were Child-Pugh class B and were more affected by smaller tumours ($P$ <0.050). Therefore, the results in terms of both patient survival and recurrence rates are biased by covariate distribution.

Results for this tumour size were published in more detail within the observational studies.

## 11.2.2 Observational Studies

One multi-institutional database of the Liver Cancer Study Group of Japan involved 2550 patients. In their report of tumours less than or equal to 2 cm, disease-free survival was significantly better after resection than after RFA ($P=0.001$, $n=1235$ vs. $n=1315$), but patient survival was similar ($P=0.280$). Therapy and Child-Pugh class were independent prognostic factors of DFS, but regression on patient survival overall was not performed. This report represents the largest series published in the literature that analysed this specific tumour size.

Wang et al. attempted to offset the different covariate distribution by matching the patients. In their subanalysis of 104 matched patients with solitary tumours ≤2 cm ($n=52$ vs. $n=52$), resection and RFA demonstrated similar patient survival ($P=0.296$), but again, DFS was significantly better in surgical patients ($P=0.031$). Despite attempting to match the patients, they later still demonstrated significantly different covariates after matching in another subset of patients ($P<0.001$), creating some doubt over the accuracy of their match procedure.

A third report, published by Peng in 2012, involved 145 with solitary tumours ≤2 cm. In this study, recurrence-free survival was unaffected ($P=0.548$); however, overall survival was better after RFA ($P=0.048$). Although not formally matched, the two groups had similar clinical and demographical covariates. Multivariate regression analyses demonstrated that treatment allocation was the only significant prognostic factor for overall survival ($P=0.046$).

It is difficult to draw definite conclusions regarding tumours of less than 2 cm, based on the lack of evidence from RCTs; however, there is some evidence that RFA can provide similar survival to that of resection. However, there does appear to be an increased recurrence rate after RFA, which is likely to be expected given the small size, and also justifies the comparable survival rates.

### Conclusion

Hepatic resection is considered the preferred treatment for patients with a single nodule or multiple lesions with good liver function, who are unsuitable for liver transplantation. Although the literature to date suggests that RFA is comparable to HR in small (<2 cm) tumours with regard to oncological outcome with a lower complication rate, the recurrence rates are much higher compared with HR. For tumour >2 cm, the overall survival in the RFA group was significantly lower than that of the HR group. As a result, it is clear that surgical resection is the treatment method for larger tumours and those patients with any complicating factors. Independent prognostic factors affecting the survival of patients include tumour size, number of lesions, location, liver function, presence of portal vein invasion, presence of vascular invasion and the width of the tumour-free margin during surgical excision. Many patients would not be eligible for randomisation due to relative or absolute contraindications to one or other treatment modality. Approximately 80 % of patients would be unsuitable for hepatic resection due to liver dysfunction and/or portal hypertension, large/multiple tumour(s), age, other co-morbidities or the location of the tumour (due to risk of extensive parenchymal damage, bleeding, peritoneal seeding or damage to other structures, such as the diaphragm). Local ablation with RFA, laser or percutaneous ethanol injection (PEI) is recommended as the standard of care for patients not suitable for surgery.

The recurrence rate after RFA is often related to incomplete tumour ablation, with the local recurrence rate differing markedly amongst patients with and without a sufficient safety margin. However, as a minimally invasive procedure, it is often hard to achieve a specific safety margin in three dimensions around large tumours, without compromising liver function, which is likely to be one of the reasons for the higher recurrence rate, but relatively low postoperative complication rate. In addition to this, it is rare for patients with small HCCs to die early on, and therefore, the recurrence only impacts on the overall survival gradually.

## 11.3  Clinical Guidelines on Management of HCC

The most recent UK guidelines were commissioned by the British Society of Gastroenterology and were published in 2003 [4]. They state that as the only potentially curative treatments, liver transplantation and hepatic resection should be offered as first-line treatments in all suitable patients. Liver resection should be the primary therapy for all those with non-cirrhotic livers. It also states that resection can be conducted in patients with cirrhosis but well-preserved liver function (Child-Pugh A), where transplantation is not possible. Nonsurgical treatments are described as options for those who are unsuitable for surgery. At the time of publication of these guidelines (2003), there were no randomised controlled trials comparing RFA to surgical resection.

## References

1. Chen MS, Li JQ, Zheng Y, Guo RP, Liang HH, Zhang YQ, et al. A prospective randomized trial comparing percutaneous local ablative therapy and partial hepatectomy for small hepatocellular carcinoma. Ann Surg. 2006;243:321–8.
2. Huang J, Yan L, Cheng Z, Wu H, Du L, Wang J, et al. A randomized trial comparing radiofrequency ablation and surgical resection for HCC conforming to the Milan criteria. Ann Surg. 2010;252:903–12.
3. Feng K, Yan J, Li X, Xia F, Ma K, Wang S, et al. A randomized controlled trial of radiofrequency ablation and surgical resection in the treatment of small hepatocellular carcinoma. J Hepatol. 2012;57:794–802.
4. Ryder SD. Guidelines for the diagnosis and treatment of hepatocellular carcinoma (HCC) in adults. Gut. 2003;52(Suppl III):iii1–8.
5. Wang Y, et al. Radiofrequency ablation versus hepatic resection for small hepatocellular carcinomas: a meta-analysis of randomized and nonrandomized controlled trials. PLoS One. 2014;9(1):e84484.

# Index

© Springer Science+Business Media Dordrecht 2016
M. Chen et al. (eds.), *Radiofrequency Ablation for Small Hepatocellular Carcinoma*,
DOI 10.1007/978-94-017-7258-7

GPSR Compliance

*The European Union's (EU) General Product Safety Regulation (GPSR) is a set of rules that requires consumer products to be  safe and our obligations to ensure this.*

*If you have any concerns about our products, you can contact us on ProductSafety@springernature.com*

In case Publisher is established outside the EU, the EU authorized representative is:

Springer Nature Customer Service Center GmbH
Europaplatz 3
69115 Heidelberg, Germany

**Batch number: 10084931**

Printed by Printforce, the Netherlands